Women's health: across age and frontier

World Health Organization
Geneva
1992

WHO Library Cataloguing in Publication Data

Women's Health : across age and frontier.

1.Women's health – statistics

ISBN 92 4 156152 1   (NLM Classification: WA 16)

The World Health Organization welcomes requests for permission to reproduce or translate its publications, in part or in full. Applications and enquiries should be addressed to the Office of Publications, World Health Organization, Geneva, Switzerland, which will be glad to provide the latest information on any changes made to the text, plans for new editions, and reprints and translations already available.

Designed by WHO Graphics
Printed in Switzerland
92/9203 Impressa

Contents

Acknowledgements

This book was prepared under the general direction of Dr A. El Bindari Hammad, Dr S. Lyagoubi-Ouahchi and Mrs N. Mahmoud Sheta, with Ms V. Hammer-Wylie of Mothercare, John Snow Inc., as principal editor.

Contributors: Ms C. AbouZahr, Dr M. Belsey, Dr D. Blake, Ms S. Cherney, Dr E. Chigan, Dr C. Chollat-Traquet, Mr T. Farkas, Dr M. Fathalla, Ms J. Ferguson, Mrs T. Gastaut, Dr K. Giri, Dr E.H.T. Goon, Dr S. Gove, Dr G. Hafez, Dr H.R. Hapsara, Dr I. Kickbusch, Dr W. Kreisel, Dr K. Lee, Dr J.C. Martines, Dr L.J. Martinez, Mrs C. Mulholland, Dr A. Petros-Barvazian, Mrs Z. Pritchard, Dr R. de los Rios, Dr J. Rochon, Ms E. Royston, Dr M. Simpson-Hebert, Ms J. Sims, Dr M. Tazaki, Dr R. Thapa, Dr J. Tulloch, Dr C. Vlassof, Administrative Committee on Coordination/Subcommittee on Nutrition, United Nations agencies such as the International Labour Organisation, the United Nations Population Fund and the United Nations Children's Fund, nongovernmental organizations such as the International Women's Health Coalition, and many others too numerous to mention.

WHO acknowledges the generous contributions received from the Carnegie Corporation of New York and the Swedish International Development Authority (SIDA) for the preparation of this book.

Introduction

The right to health is the most basic of all human rights. The Constitution of the World Health Organization asserts that:

> *"The enjoyment of the highest attainable standard of health is one of the fundamental rights of every human being without distinction of race, religion, political belief, economic or social condition."*

This means that every human being has the right to live in an environment with minimum health risks, and to have access to health services that can prevent or alleviate their suffering, treat disease, and help maintain and promote good health throughout the individual's life. Many women, wherever they live in the world, are being denied this basic human right.

This situation is a result of women's vulnerability. Their vulnerability may stem from the physical environment in which they live, their employment status, or a multitude of other factors. But in the vast majority of cases the origins of their vulnerability are found in factors specifically related to gender. While "sex" is used to refer to the biological attributes of men and women, "gender" is understood here as a social construct, referring to the distinguishing characteristics of men and women. Gender can be seen as the full range of personality traits, attitudes, feelings, values, behaviours and activities that society ascribes to the two sexes on a differential basis.

The implications of these gender differences, and the nature of the discrimination and disadvantages that women face, permeate women's social, productive and reproductive roles in all societies. The results can be seen in numerous areas. Women lag behind men on virtually every indicator of social and economic status. They constitute a larger proportion of the poor in all societies and they are relatively powerless to change the conditions of their lives – to break the bonds of poverty or to improve their health and quality of life.

In the past three decades many studies have demonstrated the importance of women's health. It is now accepted that women's health status has an important impact on the health of their children, the family, the community and the environment. And yet, despite these assertions, and despite the rapid technological advances that have been made in a number of fields, many women still suffer from preventable morbidity and mortality. While some improvements have been recorded in physical quality-of-life indicators, the health status of women remains precarious and, in some situations, is worsening. This is the human rights drama.

This book makes no attempt to address all aspects of sociopolitical and economic development affecting women's lives. A few indicators have been selected as illustrative of the socioeconomic determinants of the health of women, such as literacy, participation in the labour force and unemployment. While income levels, educational levels and life expectancy are good indicators of the outcome of development strategies, in the final analysis these and other aspects of the development process – whether positive or negative – are reflected in health status.

Numerous conferences, meetings and symposia have focused on aspects of women's health. They have been useful in that they have highlighted and made visible many of the most important health problems of women. Many of these meetings have adopted resolutions and guidelines for action, which have led to the disaggregation of data and to programmes being established aimed at improving the health of women worldwide. One example is the Safe Motherhood Initiative, launched in 1987 as a global effort to reduce maternal mortality and morbidity. Much of the information generated has provided a growing body of evidence about how social, political and economic inequities are ultimately reflected in women's health status.

Analysis of data by sex and age has allowed the separation of health issues into those related to biological sex differences and those that arise as a result of the social construct of gender. The gender factor permeates all aspects of women's health, influencing morbidity and mortality among women, research on women-specific health problems, disease transmission, especially with regard to sexually transmitted diseases and HIV infection, treatment of disease, the social stigma attached to certain health conditions, and the social and economic implications of diseases such as AIDS and malaria.

This is not to say that all is known. On the contrary, much of the work that has been done and the data that are available serve to emphasize that the "gender factor" has been missed in many areas, and that many important questions require a new kind of investigation.

This book attempts to highlight certain health outcomes of the inequity and discrimination in a series of visual presentations, covering the lifespan of women from before birth to death. Women's lifespan has been chosen as the focus for a number of reasons:

- Intergenerational health effects. Deficiencies in early life affect women's health and reproductive performance and that of their daughters.
- The importance of adolescence. Adolescence is a critical time in a woman's physical and mental development. Many lifestyle and behaviour patterns and practices established at this time influence the rest of her life, her own health and that of her family and children.
- The importance of viewing women's reproduction within the broader context. Safe motherhood cannot be seen in isolation from broader concerns of women's nutrition, education, work, and life as a whole.

- The significance of elderly women. Women account for the majority of the elderly population and this trend is increasing. The emerging health problems of the elderly in all societies have important implications for development policies and health care considerations.

The data in this book have been compiled from diverse sources. It is important to note that data that are not available are as revealing as those that are. It is known, for example, that tropical diseases such as onchocerciasis probably affect equal numbers of men and women and yet the available data show lower incidence among women. What is not being shown by these data is that there may be deliberate under-reporting by women because of the social ostracism that they may suffer as a result of the disease. It is just beginning to be understood that women who suffer from this or other similar diseases may be shunned by the community, considered unfit for marriage, and even banished from the community to die alone. When faced with this, many women may try to hide the symptoms of disease as long as possible or seek treatment secretly.

The facts and figures presented in this book, together with the photographs, provide a vivid account of women's health problems and provide the context for many more that are not covered here. Topics such as service coverage, the role of women as health care providers, the participation of women's organizations in health care, and the roles of women providing health care in the home, although very important, have not been considered.

Nevertheless, many questions are raised regarding the implications of women's health needs for health services. Questions relate to a range of issues including distance, cost, supplies and equipment, and highlight the importance of viewing services from a woman's perspective. There are women's dimensions in all aspects of expansion and reorganization of services, and analysis of access and quality of care. For example, questions concern:

■ Social and economic determinants of women's use of services: various cultural, religious, and financial factors constitute constraints to women's access to health services or health education; there are problems linked with women's low self-esteem, lack of awareness that the pain and fatigue they accept as "their lot" may be symptoms of chronic and potentially fatal conditions; women's time constraints and workload inhibit their use of services.

■ Implications for the content of health care: the woman's perspective implies an integration of services with attention to women's needs throughout the life cycle, and with integration and expansion of reproductive health care as a whole, including obstetric care, family planning, treatment of reproductive tract infections and sexually transmitted diseases, breast care, cervical cancer detection and treatment, etc. The integration of services also means that all aspects of health services are incorporated so that attention is given in a timely manner.

■ The quality of care: criteria to evaluate quality of care need to address women's issues, including health service utilization and content aspects referred to above, women's satisfaction with services, and the extent to which women's views are taken into account.

■ Training and deployment of health personnel: there is a need to examine how health personnel are sensitized to women's issues; to devise methods for improving interactions between health providers and women, with attention to counselling techniques and information provision; to overcome constraints on increasing the numbers of female doctors and other health personnel in all domains.

Women's health is viewed as a continuum. The book starts with socioeconomic determinants and then follows women's lifespan, showing the effects on female morbidity and mortality of discrimination during childhood; the significance of reproduction, and alcohol and drug use in adolescence; the health risks and problems inherent in women's work and time use; the importance of maternal health problems; the complexity of the problems associated with major diseases and infections; the seriousness of violence against women and mental disorders; and the emerging health problems of elderly women.

The reasons that women suffer from illness, disease, and pain are numerous and complex. Solutions to problems must take account of this reality. Concentrating on individual causes is misleading since it ignores the many interrelated factors that make up the life of girls and women and are reflected in their health status. It is hoped that this book will help spur actions that focus on the strategies required to improve women's health throughout the world.

Socioeconomic determinants

- Women's status
- Female literacy and population growth
- Infant mortality and female literacy, by income level
- Mothers' education and preventive health care
- Health status of women in various regions
- Regional distribution of female labour force and its increase over time
- Female–male gaps
- Women's lagging wages
- Percentage of female-headed households
- Percentage of births to unmarried women

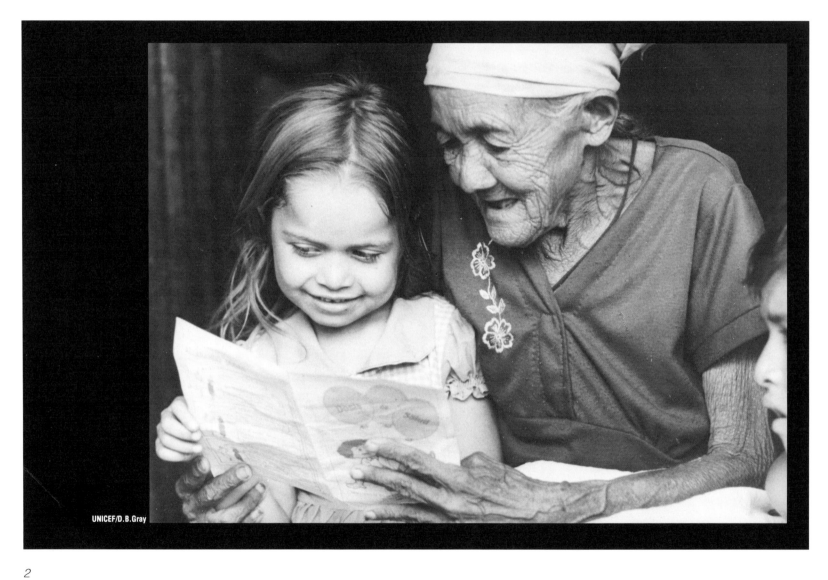

UNICEF/D.B.Gray

Women's status

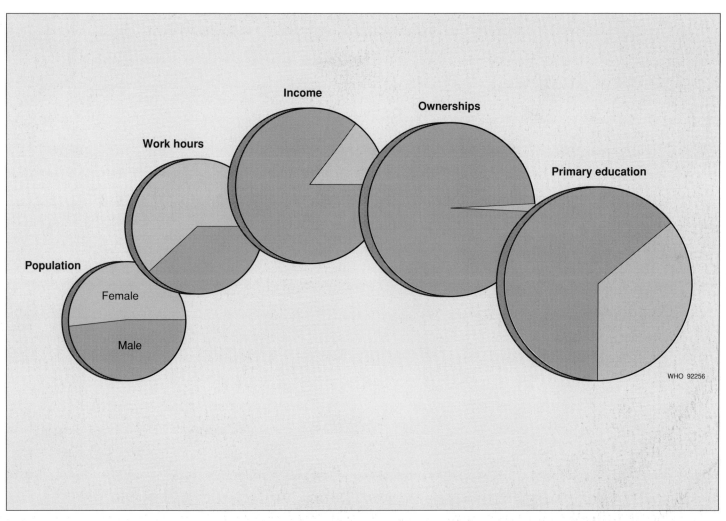

Population

Female

Male

Work hours

Income

Ownerships

Primary education

WHO 92256

Source: Kickbusch I et al. *Healthy Public Policy: Report on the Adelaide Conference.* 2nd International
Conference on Health Promotion, Adelaide, 5-9 April 1988, p. 5.

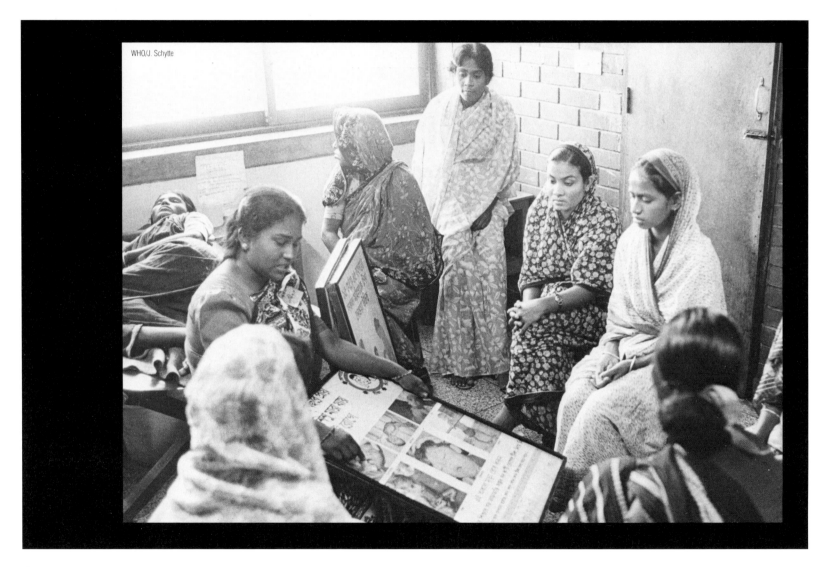

Female literacy and population growth

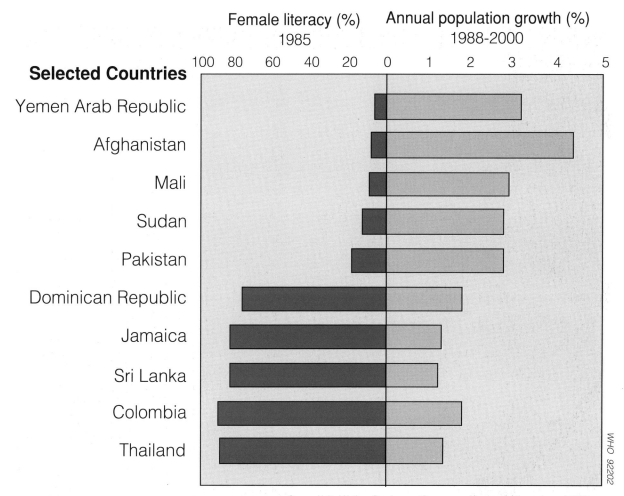

Female literacy (%)
1985

Annual population growth (%)
1988-2000

Source: United Nations Development Programme. *Human development report 1990*,
New York, Oxford University Press, 1990, p. 31.

Infant mortality by national income level and female literacy rate, around 1980

Infant mortality rate (per 1000 live births)

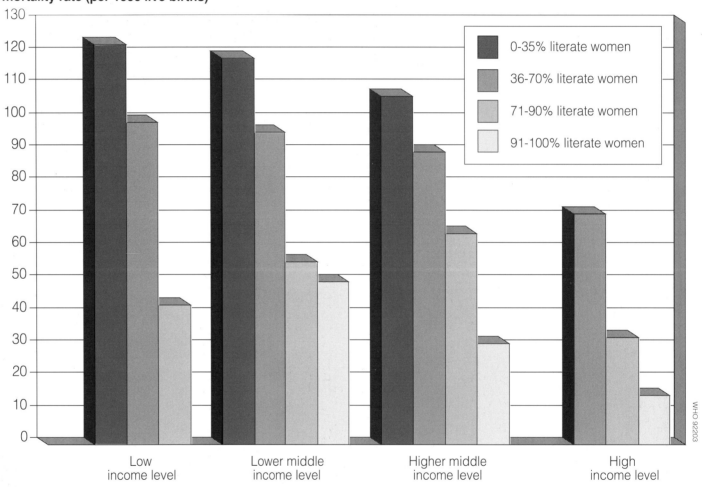

Legend:
- 0-35% literate women
- 36-70% literate women
- 71-90% literate women
- 91-100% literate women

Low income level · Lower middle income level · Higher middle income level · High income level

WHO 92203

Source: *World health statistics annual 1985.* Geneva, World Health Organization, 1986, p.10.

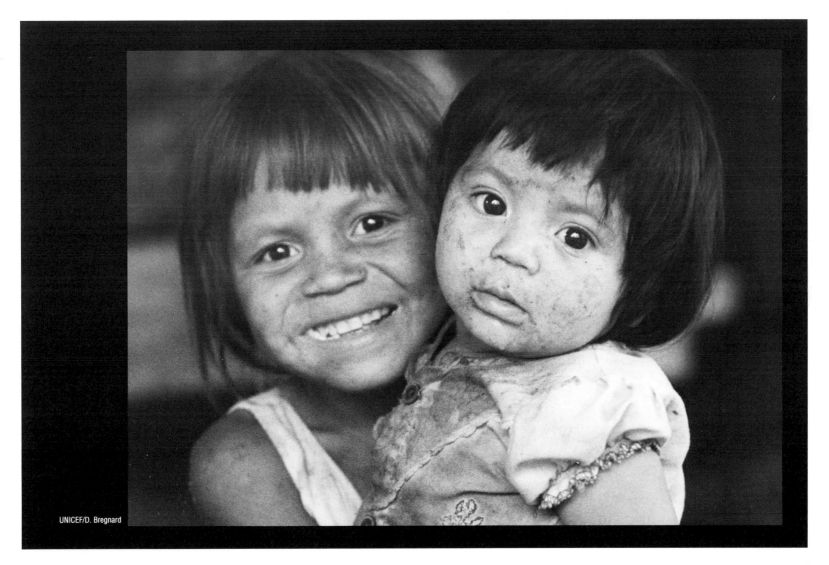

UNICEF/D. Bregnard

Mothers' education and preventive health care, around 1980

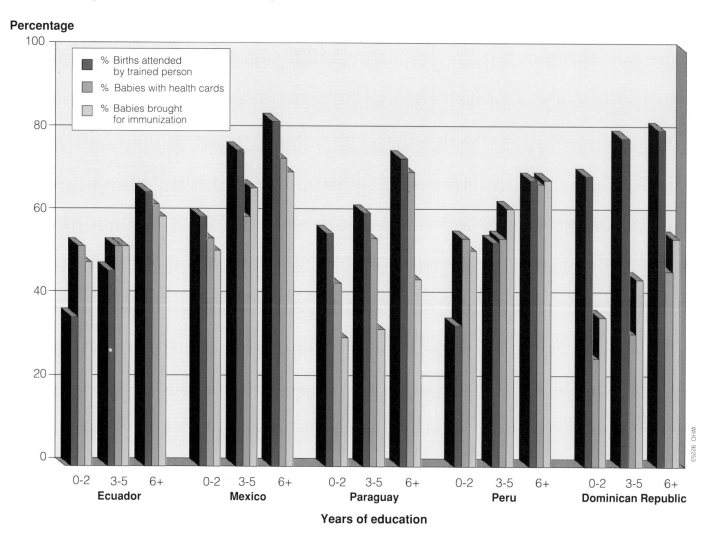

Percentage

% Births attended
by trained person

% Babies with health cards

% Babies brought
for immunization

Ecuador   **Mexico**   **Paraguay**   **Peru**   **Dominican Republic**

0-2   3-5   6+

Years of education

WHO 92253

Source: Sadik N. *Investing in women: the focus of the '90s.* New York, United Nations Population Fund (undated), p. 22.

Health status of women in various regions

Region	Life expectancy at birth (years) 1985–90[1]	Maternal mortality per 100 000 live births 1988[2]	Incidence of low birth weight %[3]	% women aged 15 - 49 with haemoglobin below normal[4]		
				Pregnant <11g/dl	Non-pregnant <12g/dl	All women
Asia	64	380	20	59	44	45
Africa	54	630	15	51	40	42
Latin America	70	200	11	41	30	34
Developed countries	77	26	7	17	12	12

Sources:
(1) *UN World Population Prospects 1990.* New York, United Nations, Department of International Economic and Social Affairs, 1991.
(2) New estimates of maternal mortality. *Weekly epidemiological record,* 1991, 66(47):346.
(3) Ghassemi H. Women, food and nutrition - issues in need of a global focus. In: *Women and nutrition.* ACC/SCN Symposium Report. Geneva, United Nations Administrative Committee on Coordination - Subcommittee on Nutrition, 1990 (Nutrition Policy Discussion Paper No. 6) p. 147.
(4) *Prevalence of nutritional anaemia in women in the world.* Geneva, World Health Organization, 1992 (unpublished document WHO/MCH/MSM/92.2).

Women's nutrition is a critical part of their overall health status. It is related among other things, to food intake during their lifetime, the nourishment they received before birth, their energy output and workload, their control over resources for household food security, and their roles in the food chain.

Regional distribution of female labour force and its increase over time

Region	Female labour force		% Increase during 1975 - 1985
	No. (millions)	Percentage	
World	676	100	8.4
Asia	382	56.5	9
Africa	61	9.0	11.2
Latin America	33	4.9	19.5
North America	46	6.5	8
Europe	151	22.3	—

Source: Ghassemi H. Women, food and nutrition - issues in need of a global focus. In: *Women and nutrition.* ACC/SCN Symposium Report. Geneva, United Nations Administrative Committee on Coordination – Subcommittee on Nutrition, 1990 (Nutrition Policy Discussion Paper No. 6), p. 154.

Female–male gaps, 1987–1988

Women's lagging wages, mid 1980s

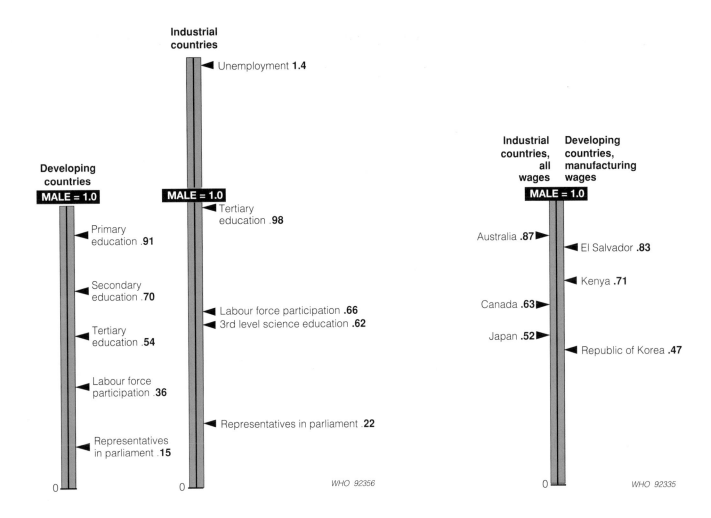

**Industrial
countries**

◀ Unemployment **1.4**

**Developing
countries**

`MALE = 1.0`

`MALE = 1.0`

◀ Tertiary
education **.98**

◀ Primary
education **.91**

◀ Secondary
education **.70**

◀ Labour force participation **.66**
◀ 3rd level science education **.62**

◀ Tertiary
education **.54**

◀ Labour force
participation **.36**

◀ Representatives in parliament **.22**

◀ Representatives
in parliament **.15**

0

0

WHO 92356

**Industrial
countries,
all
wages**

**Developing
countries,
manufacturing
wages**

`MALE = 1.0`

Australia **.87** ▶

◀ El Salvador **.83**

◀ Kenya **.71**

Canada **.63** ▶

Japan **.52** ▶

◀ Republic of Korea **.47**

0

WHO 92335

Source: United Nations Development Programme, Human development report 1991, New York, Oxford University Press, p. 30, p. 33.

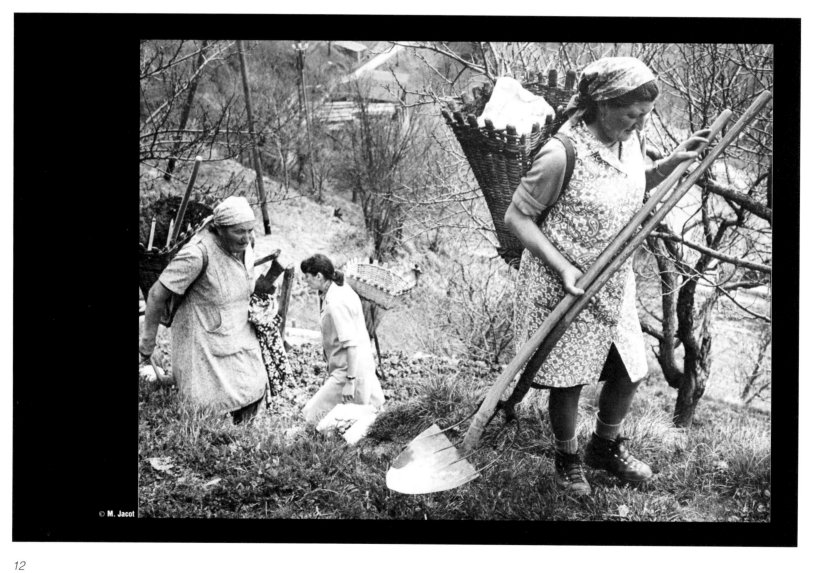

© M. Jacot

Percentage of female-headed households, 1980s

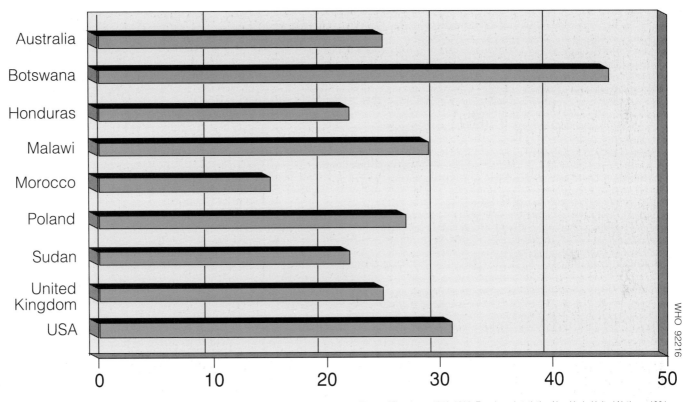

Source: Abstracted from *The world's women 1970-1990. Trends and statistics.* New York, United Nations, 1991
(Social Statistics and Indicators, Series K, No. 8), p. 18.

Households headed by women are the most economically disadvantaged.
The growing numbers of these households and of single-parent families will
aggravate conditions of poverty in both developed and developing countries.
What are the health patterns in such households? Do the trends indicate a
deterioration in health status for women and children?

Percentage of births to unmarried women, 1970 and 1985

	1970	1985
Developed regions		
Australia	8	16
Austria	13	22
Bulgaria	9	11
Denmark	11	43
Finland	6	16
German Democratic Republic	13	34
France	7	20
New Zealand	13	25
Norway	7	26
Portugal	7	12
Sweden	18	46
United Kingdom	8	19
United States	10	21
Africa		
Mauritius	3	26
Reunion	24	44
Seychelles	45	70

	1970	1985
Latin America and Caribbean		
Argentina	26	33
Bahamas	29	62
Belize	44	54
Chile	20	32
Costa Rica	29	37
French Guiana	63	76
Guadeloupe	43	57
Martinique	51	64
Puerto Rico	19	27
Asia and Pacific		
Guam	9	30
Hong Kong	3	6
Philippines	3	6

Note: Years are approximate.

Source: Abstracted from *The world's women 1970-1990. Trends and statistics.* New York, United Nations, 1991 (Social Statistics and Indicators, Series K, No. 8), p. 16.

Infancy and childhood

■ Preference for the sex of children

■ Breast-feeding and weaning practices, Bahrain, Oman, Tunisia

■ Sex-specfic incidence rates for ARI and LRI

■ Sex distribution of inpatients and outpatients

■ Child nutrition by sex and household status, Punjab, India

■ Sex-specific mortality and sex mortality ratio (M/F) for selected groups of causes of death among children aged 1 to 4

■ Annual death rate among 2-5-year-olds, by sex

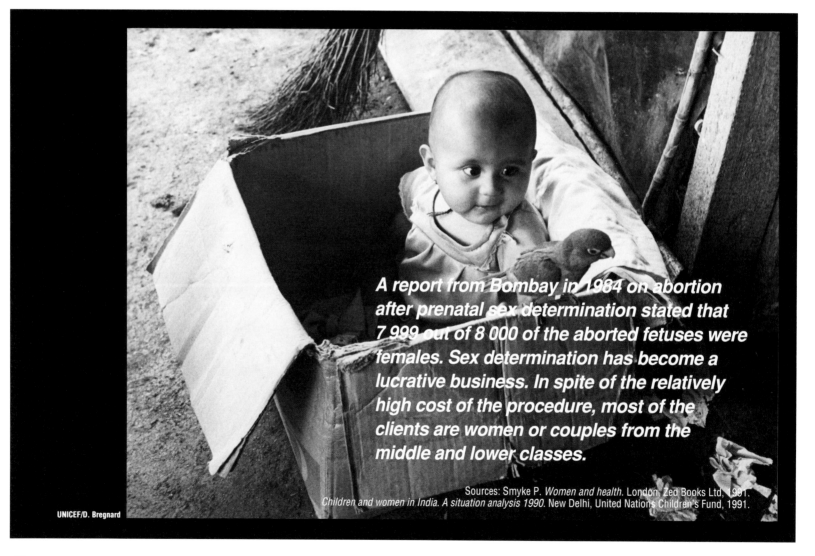

A report from Bombay in 1984 on abortion after prenatal sex determination stated that 7 999 out of 8 000 of the aborted fetuses were females. Sex determination has become a lucrative business. In spite of the relatively high cost of the procedure, most of the clients are women or couples from the middle and lower classes.

Sources: Smyke P. *Women and health*. London, Zed Books Ltd, 1991.
Children and women in India. A situation analysis 1990. New Delhi, United Nations Children's Fund, 1991.

UNICEF/D. Bregnard

Preference for the sex of children

Country	Index of son preference
Strong son preference	
Pakistan	4.9
Nepal	4.0
Bangladesh	3.3
Republic of Korea	3.3
Syrian Arab Republic	2.3
Jordan	1.9

Country	Index of son preference
Moderate son preference	
Egypt	1.5
Lesotho	1.5
Senegal	1.5
Sri Lanka	1.5
Sudan	1.5
Thailand	1.4
Turkey	1.4
Fiji	1.3
Nigeria	1.3
Tunisia	1.3
Yemen Arab Republic	1.3
Cameroon	1.2
Dominican Republic	1.2
Côte d'Ivoire	1.2
Malaysia	1.2
Mexico	1.2
Morocco	1.2

Country	Index of son preference
No preference	
Guyana	1.1
Indonesia	1.1
Kenya	1.1
Peru	1.1
Trinidad and Tobago	1.1
Colombia	1.0
Costa Rica	1.0
Ghana	1.0
Panama	1.0
Paraguay	1.0
Portugal	1.0
Haiti	0.9
Philippines	0.9
Daughter preference	
Venezuela	0.8
Jamaica	0.7

Index of son preference = ratio of the number of mothers who prefer the next child to be male to the number of mothers who prefer the next child to be female.

Source: Royston E, Armstrong S. *Preventing maternal deaths.* Geneva, World Health Organization, 1989, p. 51.

The preference for boy babies is an almost universal phenomenon, and is closely linked with the perception of women's poor economic potential.

"One son is worth more than three daughters"
– A proverb

"Having a son is like having two eyes. Having a daughter is like having only one eye"
– A proverb

Breast-feeding and weaning practices, Bahrain, Oman, and Tunisia

Studies in these and other countries show that the duration of breast-feeding is longer for boys; some studies in Latin America show that complementary feeding is begun earlier for boys than for girls.

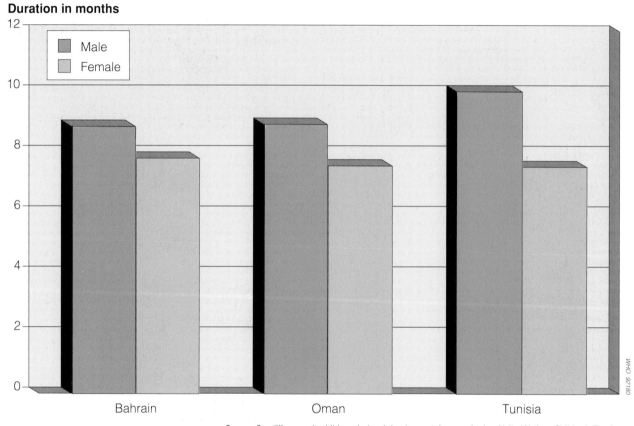

Duration in months

Legend: Male, Female

Source: *Sex differences in child survival and development.* Amman, Jordan, United Nations Children's Fund, Regional Office for the Middle East and North Africa, 1990 (Evaluation Series No. 6), p. 17.

WHO 92.181

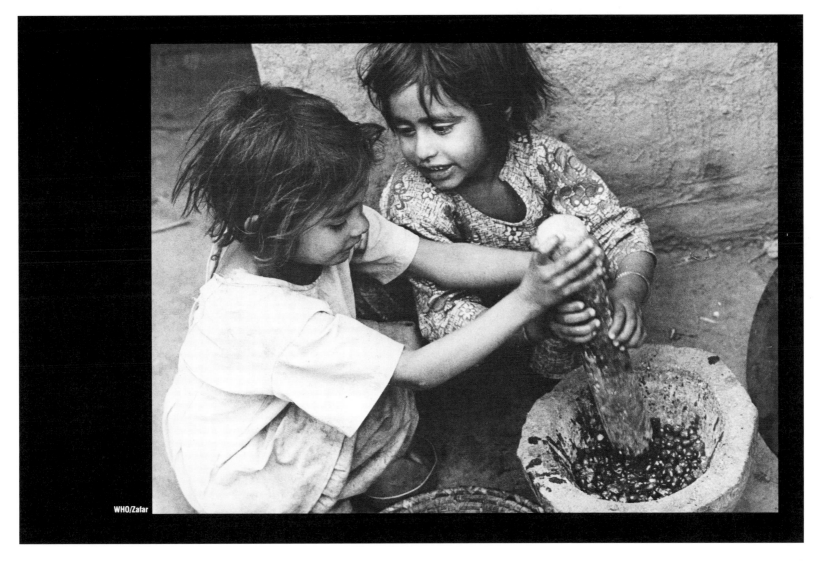

WHO/Zafar

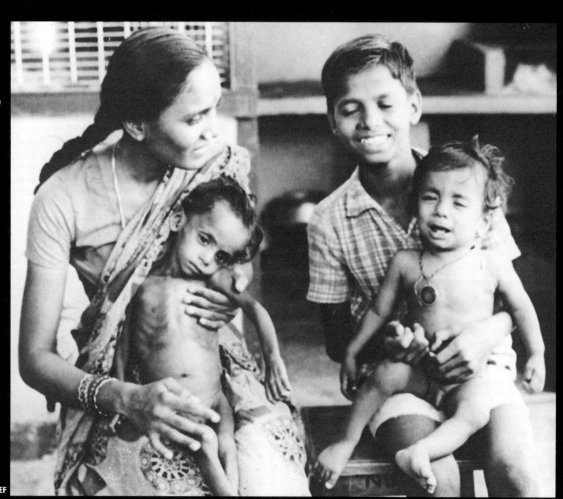

Gender discrimination is found throughout the world, from birth onwards. Research on disease prevalence, health care utilization and family resource allocation indicates that girls are treated differently from boys, with negative results that last for a lifetime.

WHO/UNICEF

Sex-specific incidence rates for ARI and LRI
per 100 child-weeks at risk in BOSTID[1] community studies

Study site	ARI Boys	ARI Girls	LRI Boys	LRI Girls
Colombia	9.8	9.7	2.9	2.1
Guatemala	17.4	16.2	0.7	0.5
Nigeria	16.1	14.8	—	—
Papua New Guinea	—	—	2.3	2.8
Philippines	13.9	13.7	1.3	1.2
Thailand	28.6	26.4	—	—
Uruguay	16.6	14.5	9.1	7.3

[1] Board on Science and Technology for International Development, National Academy of Sciences, Washington, DC

Sex distribution of inpatients and outpatients,
in BOSTID hospital studies

Type of patient, study site	URI[1] Boys (%)	URI Girls (%)	LRI Boys (%)	LRI Girls (%)
Inpatients				
Argentina	—	—	55.8	44.2
Pakistan	74.4	25.6	65.9	34.1
Philippines	—	—	55.5	44.5
Thailand	—	—	59.2	40.8
Outpatients				
Argentina	—	—	56.6	43.4
Pakistan	53.9	46.1	59.2	40.8
Thailand	62.3	37.7	54.3	45.7

[1] Upper respiratory tract infections

This study showed that the incidence rates of acute respiratory infection (ARI) and of lower respiratory tract infection (LRI) were only slightly higher for boys in community surveys, whereas many more boys than girls were found with those infections as inpatients or outpatients in hospitals.

Source: Selwyn BJ. The epidemiology of acute respiratory tract infection in young children: comparison of findings from several developing countries. *Reviews of infectious diseases*, 1990, 12 (supplement 8): S877.

Child nutrition by sex and household status, Punjab, India

Global data suggest that gender discrimination in feeding and nutritional status cuts across economic lines.

	Male %	Female %
Privileged children		
Normal nutrition	86	70
70-80% of expected weight	10	17
Less than 70% of expected weight	4	13
Underprivileged children		
Normal nutrition	43	26
70-80% of expected weight	43	24
Less than 70% of expected weight	14	50

Source: Bown L. *Preparing the future - women, literacy and development*, Chard, Somerset, ActionAid, undated (ActionAid Development Report No. 4).

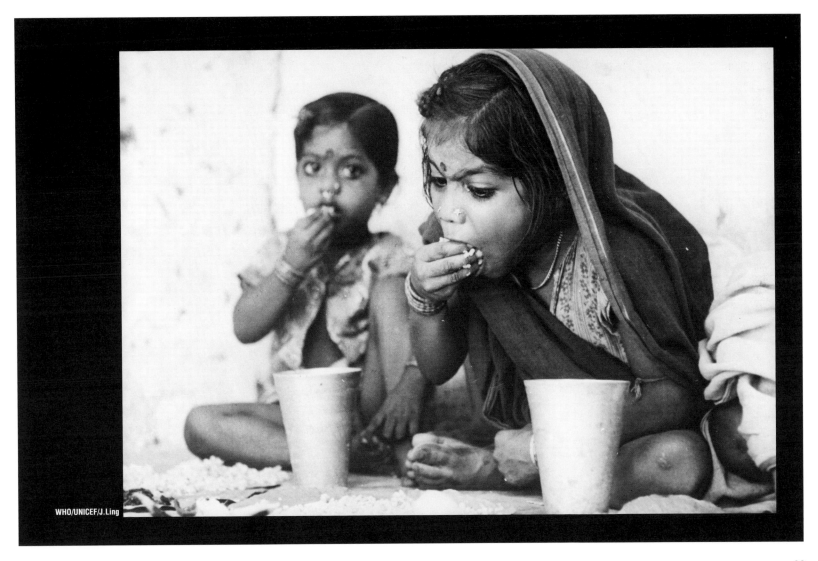

WHO/UNICEF/J.Ling

Sex-specific mortality rates and sex mortality ratio (M/F) for selected groups of causes of death among children aged 1 to 4. *Selected countries in the Americas. Most recent year with available information (rates per 100 000 population)*

Country/year	Enteritis & other diarrhoeal diseases			Acute respiratory infections			Nutritional deficiencies			Preventable by immunization			Accidents and violence		
	M	F	M/F	M	F	M/F	M	F	M/F	M	F	M/F	M	F	M/F
Canada 88	0.00	0.00	—	2.00	1.12	1.78	0.40	0.14	2.86	0.00	0.00	—	17.96	11.74	1.53
USA 88	0.07	0.04	1.59	1.65	1.60	1.03	0.36	0.28	1.29	0.00	0.00	—	26.39	18.57	1.42
Cuba 88	2.46	1.61	1.53	8.01	4.51	1.78	1.85	0.32	5.74	0.00	0.32	0.00	33.57	19.00	1.77
Costa Rica 88	10.97	4.47	2.45	8.53	8.95	0.95	0.00	1.28	0.00	0.00	0.00	—	22.55	9.58	2.35
Panama 87	30.83	20.21	1.53	23.33	19.33	1.21	15.83	18.45	0.86	3.33	8.79	0.38	24.17	21.09	1.15
Uruguay 88	3.49	0.91	3.96	5.24	5.43	0.96	0.00	0.91	0.00	0.00	0.00	—	20.94	21.72	0.96**
Chile 87	2.40	2.13	1.13	17.56	11.21	1.57	1.48	0.58	2.55	0.00	0.00	—	37.89	22.63	1.67
Argentina 86	5.49	6.45	0.85**	9.42	7.60	1.24	5.91	6.66	0.89**	0.91	1.30	0.70	29.53	19.05	1.55
Venezuela 87	18.70	17.76	1.05	18.61	19.94	0.93**	6.63	7.37	0.90**	3.18	4.54	0.70**	28.96	22.30	1.30
Mexico 86	55.97	54.02	1.04	25.89	25.14	1.03	9.38	9.09	1.03	7.13	8.71	0.82	33.08	25.40	1.30
Colombia 86	—	—	—	—	—	—	—	—	—	—	—	—	37.17	28.34	1.31
Paraguay 86	87.11	68.60	1.27	40.47	50.21	0.81**	17.15	19.10	0.90**	7.55	5.66	1.33	27.15	10.61	1.62
Dom. Rep. 85	55.41	48.92	1.13	34.46	41.27	0.84**	36.85	33.34	1.11	13.52	15.31	0.88**	16.44	10.93	1.80
Ecuador 88	87.75	87.79	1.00**	40.93	39.59	1.03	35.97	31.13	1.16	25.89	27.61	0.94**	39.54	23.14	1.71
Brazil 86	16.34	15.35	1.06	23.37	21.81	1.07	9.09	8.78	1.03	5.75	5.31	1.08	23.00	14.91	1.54
Honduras 81	114.39	94.46	1.21	28.17	25.61	1.10	14.09	24.22	0.58**	49.12	41.87	1.17	18.21	10.38	1.75
El Salvador 84	67.37	51.34	1.31	12.14	15.43	0.79**	18.21	21.10	0.86**	18.51	18.90	0.98**	17.91	12.91	1.39
Guatemala 84	340.56	349.77	0.97**	215.09	252.28	0.85**	78.15	84.84	0.92**	89.62	114.60	0.78**	15.77	7.44	2.12
Peru 83	130.07	140.21	0.93**	134.84	136.97	0.98**	45.32	47.31	0.96**	28.74	31.57	0.91	19.45	12.41	1.57

**Excess female mortality based on a total of more than 40 deaths

Source: Gomez E. *Sex discrimination and excess female mortality among children in the Americas.* Paper prepared for the 18th NCIH International Health Conference, 23-26 June 1991, Arlington, VA, p. 19.

Analysis of sex-specific mortality by cause in Latin America revealed an excess female mortality among children aged 1 to 4 years, with disproportionately more girls than boys dying from diseases preventable by immunization.

Annual death rate among 2-5-year-olds, by sex

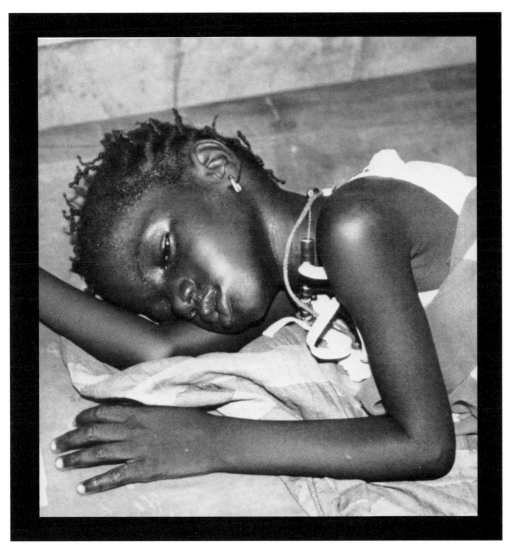

WHO/S. Lindsay

	Death rate per 1000	
	Girls	Boys
Bangladesh	68.6	57.7
Colombia	24.8	20.5
Costa Rica	8.1	4.8
Dominican Republic	20.2	17.2
Haiti	61.2	47.8
Mexico	16.7	14.7
Nepal	60.7	57.7
Pakistan	54.4	36.9
Panama	8.7	7.6
Peru	30.8	28.8
Philippines	21.9	19.1
Republic of Korea	12.7	11.8
Sri Lanka	18.7	16.3
Syrian Arab Republic	14.6	9.3
Thailand	26.8	17.3
Turkey	19.5	18.4
Venezuela	8.4	7.6

Source: *The world's women 1970-1990. Trends and statistics.*
New York, United Nations, 1991 (Social Statistics and
Indications, Series K, No. 8), p. 60.

Major long-term complications of genital mutilation include gynaecological, urinary, obstetric and marital problems. Millions of girls in many countries have undergone this procedure.

WHO/J.-C. Bruet

Adolescence

- Married youth

- Percentage of first births to women under 20 years, selected countries

- Maternal mortality by age

- Infant mortality by age of mother, Brazil

- Age-specific rates of gonorrhoea among males and females in the USA

- Distribution of smokers by sex and age in Spain

- Heavy smoking among young people, by sex

- Consumption of alcoholic drinks by young men and young women

- Daily drinking among young men and women

- Drug use by young people

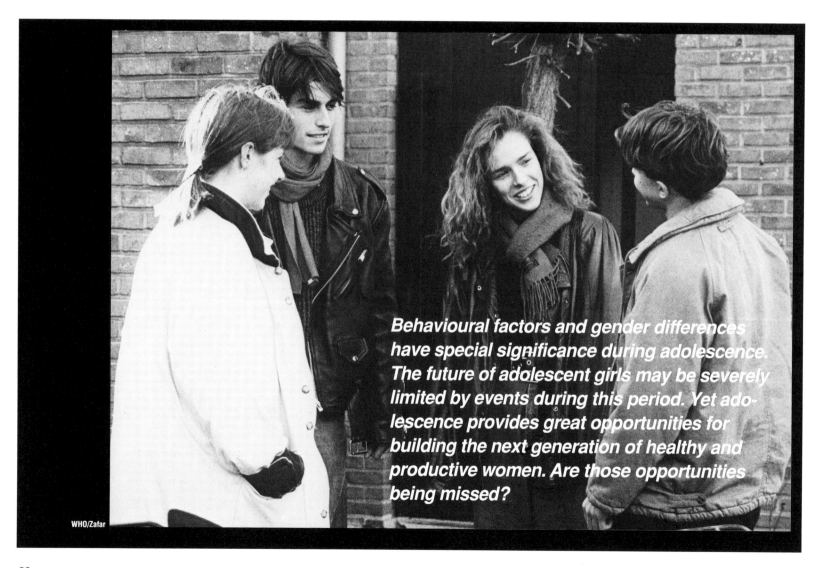

Behavioural factors and gender differences have special significance during adolescence. The future of adolescent girls may be severely limited by events during this period. Yet adolescence provides great opportunities for building the next generation of healthy and productive women. Are those opportunities being missed?

WHO/Zafar

Married youth, around 1980

Figures comparing the proportion of males and females who marry under the age of 20 illustrate vastly different life options. They imply an early start to reproduction for adolescent girls, as well as the end of educational opportunities in most countries.

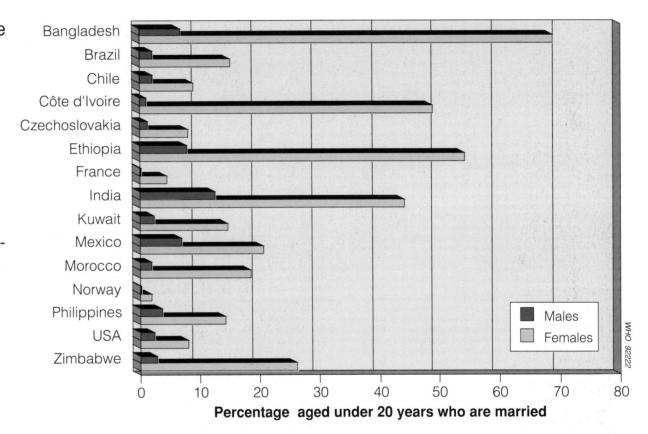

Percentage aged under 20 years who are married

WHO 92222

Source: *The health of youth. Facts for action. Youth and reproductive health.* Geneva, World Health Organization, 1989 (unpublished document A42/Technical Discussions/5), p. 2.

Demographic and health surveys show that infant mortality is highest among babies born to young mothers. To what extent does this reflect physiological immaturity only? Are other behavioural factors implicated?

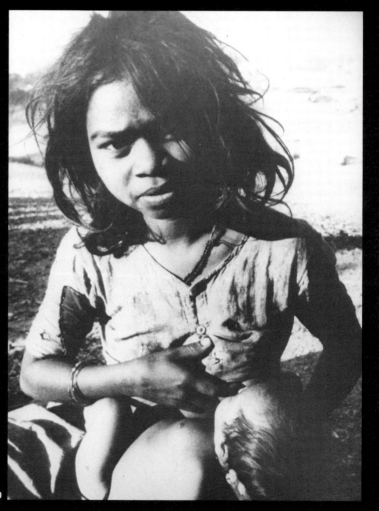

WHO/SEARO

Percentage of first births to women under 20 years, selected countries

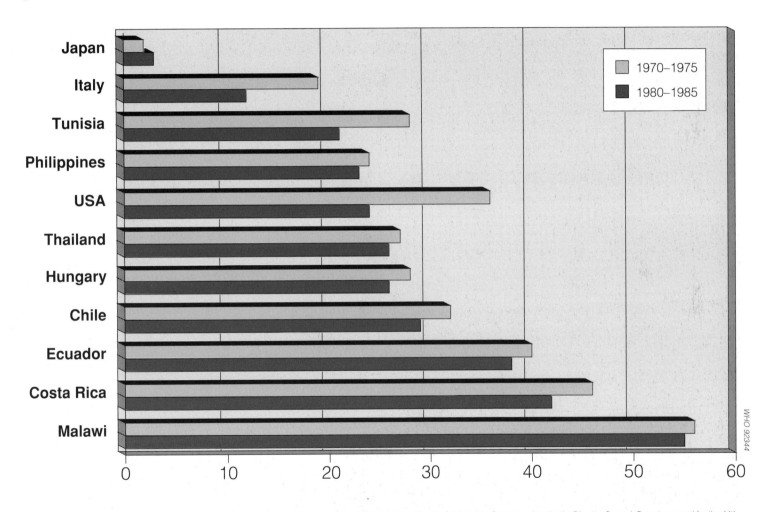

Legend:
- 1970–1975
- 1980–1985

WHO 92344

Source: *Women, health and development.* Progress report by the Director-General. Report prepared for the 44th World Health Assembly, 1991, Geneva, World Health Organization (unpublished document A44/15), p. 9.

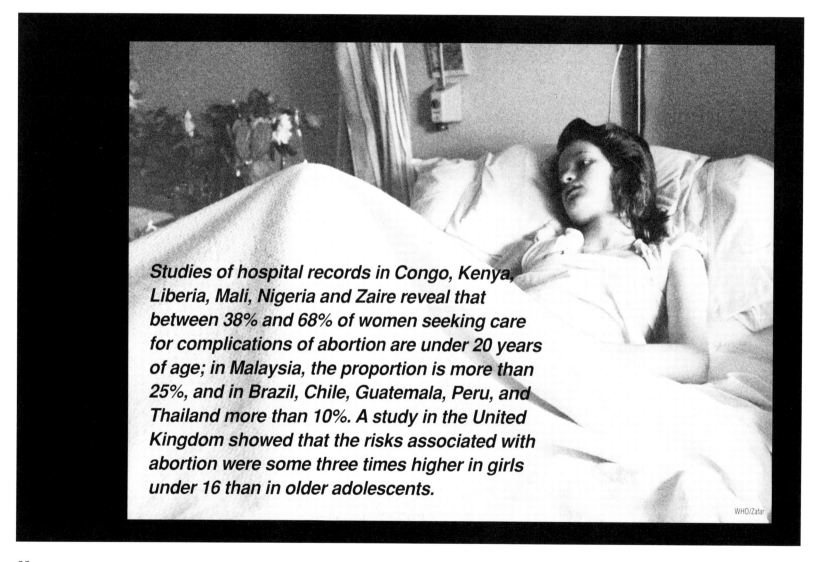

Studies of hospital records in Congo, Kenya,
Liberia, Mali, Nigeria and Zaire reveal that
between 38% and 68% of women seeking care
for complications of abortion are under 20 years
of age; in Malaysia, the proportion is more than
25%, and in Brazil, Chile, Guatemala, Peru, and
Thailand more than 10%. A study in the United
Kingdom showed that the risks associated with
abortion were some three times higher in girls
under 16 than in older adolescents.

WHO/Zafar

Maternal mortality by age, 1980s

No. of deaths per 1000 live births

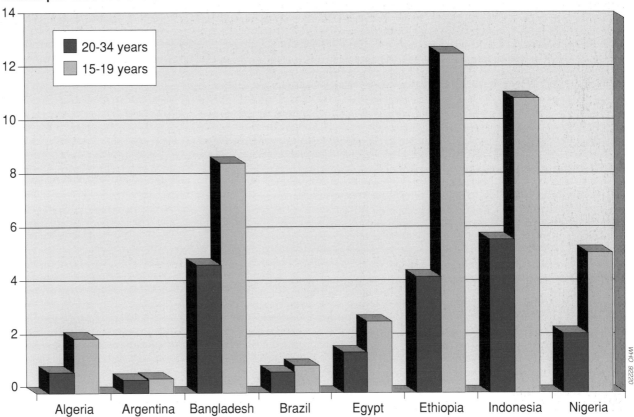

Source: *Women, health and development.* Progress report by the Director-General. Report prepared for the 44th World Health Assembly, Geneva, World Health Organization, 1991 (unpublished document A44/15), p. 8.

Data on maternal mortality by age, especially in some developing countries, underline the dangers of childbearing during early adolescence. Shouldn't health care strategies prevent these tragically premature deaths?

Infant mortality by age of mother, Brazil, 1976–86

Demographic and health surveys show that infant mortality is highest among babies born to young mothers. To what extent does this reflect physiological immaturity only? Are other behavioural factors implicated?

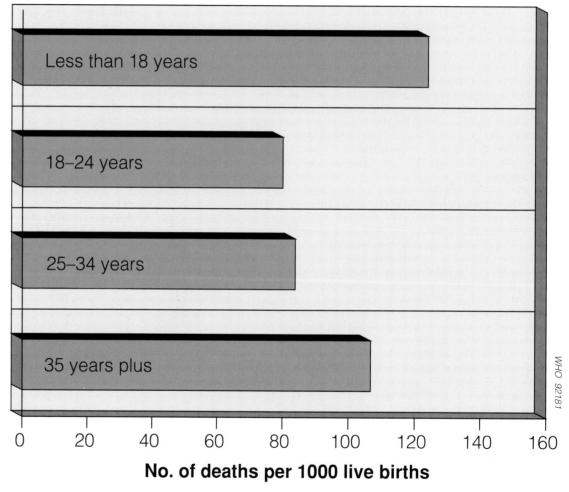

Age of mother

Less than 18 years

18–24 years

25–34 years

35 years plus

No. of deaths per 1000 live births

WHO 92181

Source: Institute for Resource Development, Demographic and Health Surveys, Columbia, Maryland. Cited in *The state of the world's children 1990*, New York, Oxford University Press for UNICEF, 1990, p. 27.

Age-specific rates of gonorrhoea among males and females in the USA, 1987

Sexually transmitted diseases (STDs) among young people are widespread and increasing. The consequences of untreated STDs include, among other things, infertility. What are the social consequences for these young women?

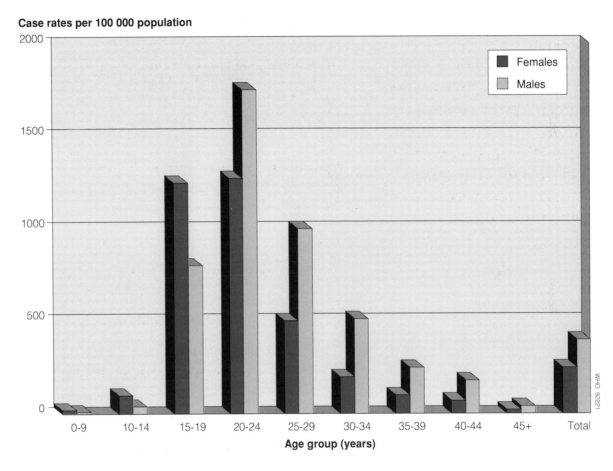

Case rates per 100 000 population

Legend: Females, Males

Age group (years): 0-9, 10-14, 15-19, 20-24, 25-29, 30-34, 35-39, 40-44, 45+, Total

WHO 92221

Source: De Schryver A, Meheus A. Epidemiology of sexually transmitted diseases: the global picture.
Bulletin of the World Health Organization, 1990, 68(5): 639-654.

Distribution of smokers by sex and age in Spain, 1987

% smokers 16 years and older

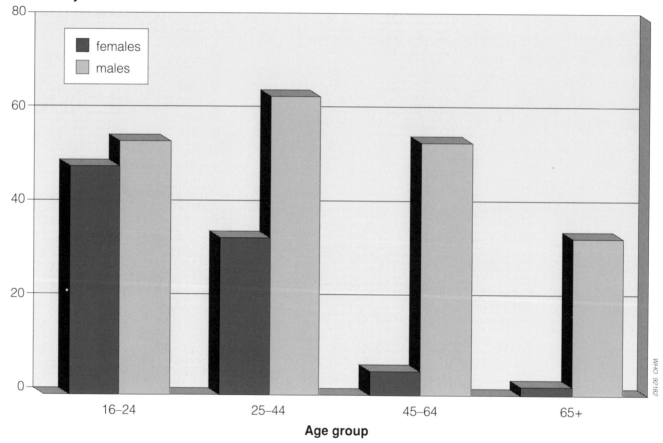

Source: National Health Survey, 1987, Cited in *Women and tobacco.* Geneva, World Health Organization, 1992, p.16.

The sex and age distribution of smokers in Spain reflects changing patterns in a rapidly "modernizing" society, putting young women at high risk.

Heavy smoking among young people, by sex

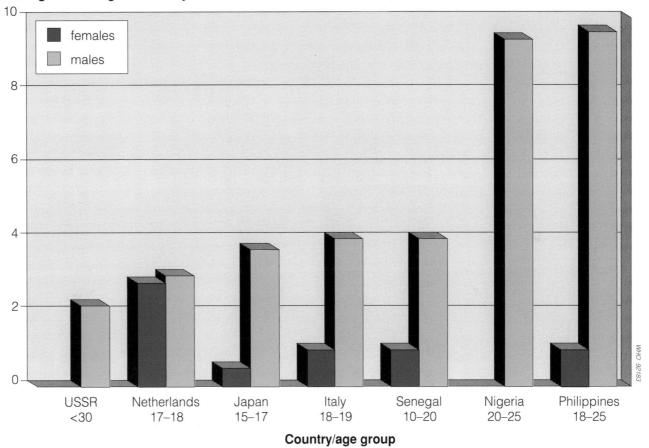

% smoking over 20 cigarettes daily

Legend:
- ■ females
- □ males

Country/age group:
- USSR <30
- Netherlands 17–18
- Japan 15–17
- Italy 18–19
- Senegal 10–20
- Nigeria 20–25
- Philippines 18–25

Country/age group

WHO 92183

Source: *Women and tobacco.* Geneva, World Health Organization, 1992, p.18

How different will the figures be in a few years if trends towards increased smoking among adolescent girls continue, and if advertising is targeted towards this group?

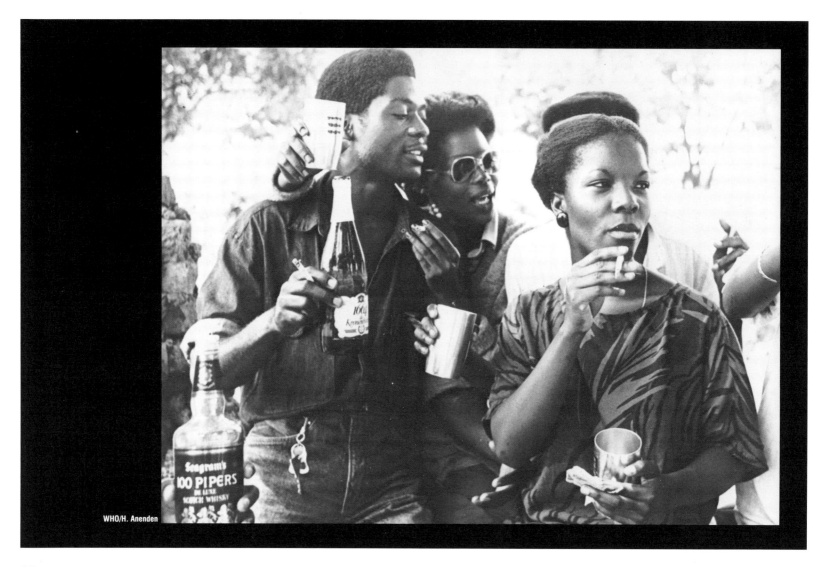

WHO/H. Anenden

Consumption of alcoholic drinks by young men and young women, by specific age group, around 1985

Developed countries/age groups

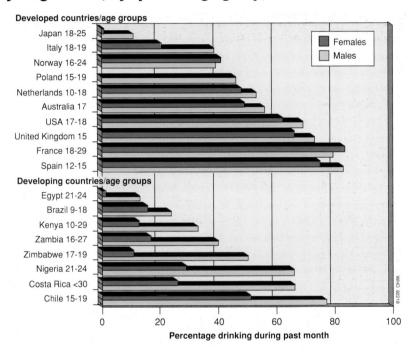

Percentage drinking during past month

Daily drinking among young men and women, around 1985

Percentage drinking every day

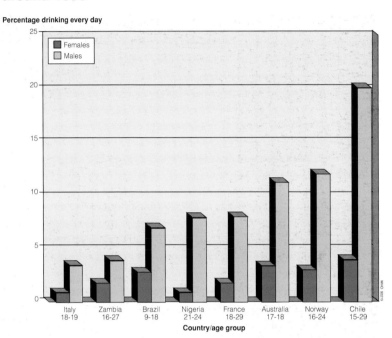

Country/age group

Source: *The health of youth. Facts for action. Youth and alcohol.* Geneva, World Health Organization, 1989 (unpublished document A42/Technical Discussions/4), p.4

Alcohol consumption among young men is generally greater than among young women, though in many countries the differences are not large. Will the situation change in the future?

Drug use by young people, Sweden, 1983

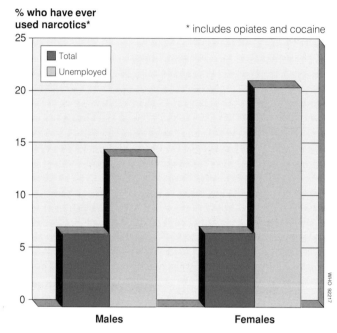

% who have ever used narcotics*

* includes opiates and cocaine

- ■ Total
- ▨ Unemployed

WHO 92217

Males   **Females**

Source: Hammarstrom A. Youth unemployment and ill-health: results from a 2-year follow-up study. *Social science and medicine*, 1988, 26(10).

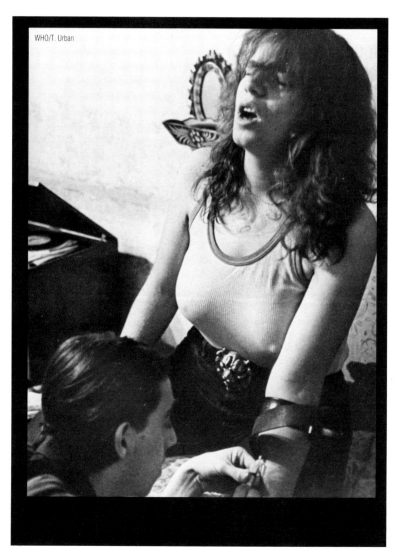

WHO/T. Urban

Substance abuse among young women is a growing concern, since the figures are increasing in both developed and developing countries. The implications for both women and men are potentially devastating but the problem has an added catastrophic dimension for young women having a baby. In New York City, the increasing number of babies born with drug dependence horrifies the medical world.

Women at work

- Work input by women and men in African agriculture

- Number employed in the large employment systems in India

- Women's contribution to household income

- Labour force participation by relationship to household head, Brazil and USA

- Primary child care arrangements in 1985 for children under 5 whose mothers work outside the home

- Nutritional intake of working women and housewives as a percentage of the recommended dietary allowance, Bombay, India

- Prevalence of chronic bronchitis in Nepalese hill villages

- Percentages of females in various age groups affected by cor pulmonale, New Delhi

- Proportion of men and women who collect water, by age, Kenya

- Incidence of selected cancers in women in mining districts compared with those in non-mining districts of Czechoslovakia

- Blood lead in children and mothers in various places within Katowice Region, Poland

Contrary to past perceptions of women as economically dependent, and of men as the breadwinners of the family, research carried out over the past 15 years provides detailed evidence of the significance of women's productive roles. It shows the need to break down artificial divisions of work, both within and outside the home. This raises questions about how gender differences in health risks and disease prevalence relate to working conditions, as well as to availability of health information and service approaches.

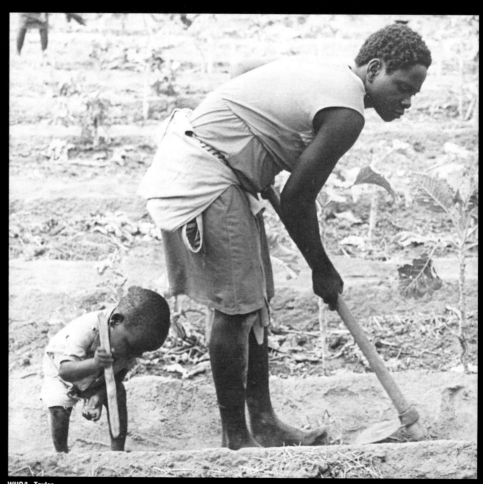

WHO/L. Taylor

Study results emphasize how vulnerable a woman's economic status can be, and how critical it is for the family as a whole. The "feminization of poverty" is the catch-phrase that describes this vulnerability. How is this translated into relationships between poverty and health? What are the gender distinctions that are hidden behind global statistics?

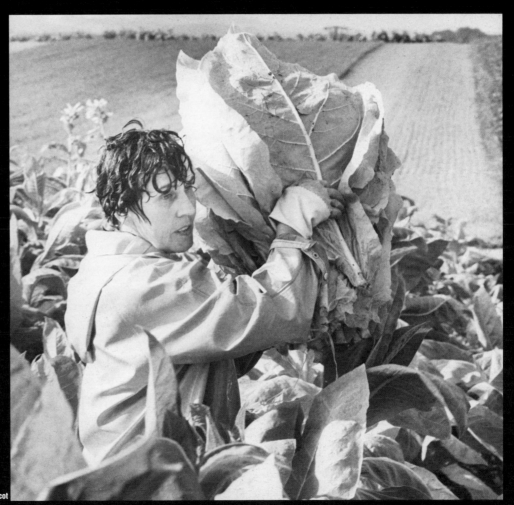

© M. Jacot

Work input by women and men in African agriculture

Country in which sample villages are located	% of women in family labour force in agriculture	Female working hours as percentage of male working hours	% of work on farm performed by family members	
			Female	Male
Cameroon	62	81	56	44
Central African Republic	58	150	68	32
Congo	57	160	68	32
Gambia	52	213	70	30
Nigeria	57	15	9	49
Senegal	53	53	29	66
Uganda	53	163	56	19

Source: abstracted from McGuire J, Popkin BM. Beating the zero sum game: women and nutrition in the Third World. In: *Women and nutrition.* ACC/SCN Symposium Report. Geneva, United Nations Administrative Committee on Coordination - Subcommittee on Nutrition, 1990, (Nutrition Policy Discussion Paper No. 6), p. 17.

Research on agricultural production documents women's heavy workload. The unpaid household work that women are responsible for adds to their working day.

Number employed in the large employment systems in India

	Women	Men
	Thousands	
Agriculture	1 900	75 600
Dairy farming	75 000	5 000
Fisheries	1 000	1 800
Small animal husbandry	15 000	2 000
Khadi & village crafts	1 700	2 000
Handicrafts	500	2 200
Sericulture	800	1 200
Handlooms	3 000	4 500

Source: Bajaj S. Nutrition security system at household level: policy implications. In: *Women and nutrition.* ACC/SCN Symposium Report. Geneva, United Nations Administrative Committee on Coordination - Subcommittee on Nutrition, 1990 (Nutrition Policy Discussion Paper No. 6), p. 125.

Women's contribution to household income

Country study*	Percentage of household income contributed by women
Cameroon, 1974	58.1
Lebanon, 1984	10
Pakistan, 1975-76	17.6
Philippines, 1975	42
Chile, 1983	
With children under 6 years	
Employed housewife	24
Unemployed housewife	28
Without children under 6 years	
Employed housewife	15
Unemployed housewife	18

* Studies listed in source.

Source: McGuire J, Popkin BM. Beating the zero sum game: women and nutrition in the Third World. In: *Women and nutrition.* ACC/SCN Symposium Report. Geneva, United Nations Administrative Committee on Coordination – Subcommittee on Nutrition (Nutrition Policy Discussion Paper No. 6), 1990, p. 20.

Labour force participation by relationship to household head, Brazil and USA

Brazil 1985

50.0% female heads of household working in labour force

32.9% wives with husband living at home

36.8% daughters

26.1% female relatives

USA 1987

56.7% unmarried women in labour force

56.1% married women in labour force

Primary child care arrangements in 1985 for children under age 5 whose mothers work outside the home

	Brazil	USA
Preschool/Centre-based care	20.4	23.9
Maid or nanny	11.1	5.9
Other paid care-giver in the care-giver's home	2.4	26.8
Unpaid care-giver in the care-giver's home	2.4	—
Grandparent in the grandparent's home	7.3	10.2
Siblings	9.8	—
Other unpaid care-giver in the child's home	9.9	9.4
Parents	36.2	23.8
Other	0.5	—
Total	**100.0**	**100.0**

Source: Connelly R, DeGraff DS, Levison D. *Child care policy and women's market work in urban Brazil.* Geneva, International Labour Office, 1991 (Population and Labour Policies Programme, Working Paper No. 180), p. 6, p. 31.

This study in Brazil is one of several that have investigated child care arrangements in situations where the mothers are working outside the home. Much more information is needed on women's coping strategies. Who is taking care of the children? What is the quality of the care being provided? Why do responsibilities for child care usually fall solely on women? What are the cost implications? What are the social and economic consequences for society as a whole?

Nutritional intake of working women and housewives as a percentage of the recommended dietary allowance, Bombay, India

Very few studies show the direct health effects of women's heavy workload. One study, carried out in India, compared women working outside the home with women working in the home in urban areas. None of the women had adequate nutritional intake and all had symptoms of nutritional deficiency. Women working outside the home fared worse in both aspects. This conclusion was confirmed in a similar study in Calcutta.

Nutritional intake as % of recommended allowance

	Working women	Housewives
Protein	78.4	84.2
Fat	73.3	70.0
Carbohydrates	65.6	86.9
Calories	66.9	84.0
Calcium	59.0	55.6
Iron	82.2	86.6
Vitamin A	17.0	12.5
Vitamin B_1 (Thiamine)	105.4	127.0
Vitamin B_2 (Riboflavin)	50.8	64.5
Vitamin B_3 (Niacin)	75.3	160.0
Vitamin C	47.5	101.5

Source: Khan ME, Tamang AK, Patel B. Work pattern of women and its impact on health and nutrition - some observations from the urban poor. *Journal of family welfare*, 1990, 36(2): 9.

Senapati SK. *Women's work pattern and its impact on health and nutrition.* Paper prepared for the 18th NCIH International Health Conference, 23-26 June 1991, Arlington, VA, p. 14.

Studies of work patterns of men and women reveal differences in exposure to health hazards. Certain health hazards are particularly linked with women's roles, such as the burning of biomass fuels used in cooking and heating inside homes, the carrying of heavy loads of water or firewood, and the use of house-hold chemicals. Toxicological effects on the fetus have also been shown. Have occupational health programmes identified and taken into account these risks? Have policies and strategies been formulated in the light of gender differences?

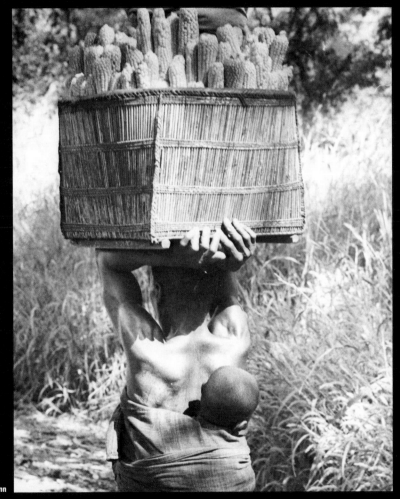

WHO/E. Mandelmann

Prevalence of chronic bronchitis in Nepalese hill villages, around 1984
Self-reported hours per day spent near cooking/heating stove

Proximity to household stoves has been linked to increased prevalence of chronic bronchitis. In most parts of the world women spend more time than men cooking indoors, and are thus at higher risk.

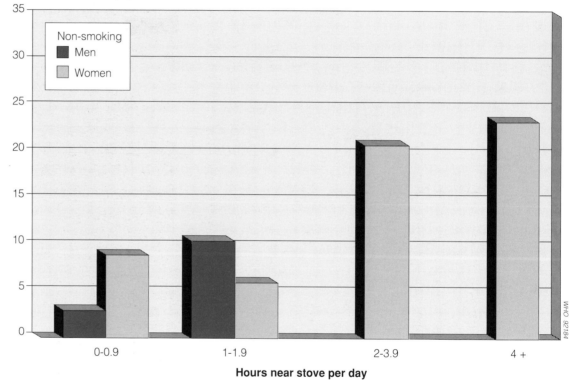

Prevalence of bronchitis (%)

Non-smoking
■ Men
■ Women

Hours near stove per day

WHO 92184

Source: Chen BH et al. Indoor air pollution in developing countries. *World health statistics quarterly*, 1990, 43(3): 130.

Percentage of females in various age groups affected by cor pulmonale, New Delhi

Prevalence of cor pulmonale (%)

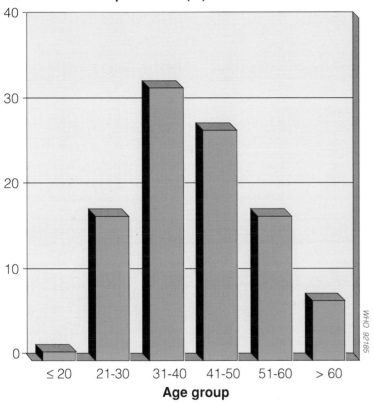

Age group

Source: Adapted from Smith KR. *Biofuels, air pollution and health - a global review.*
New York, Plenum Press, 1987, p. 208.

WHO 92185

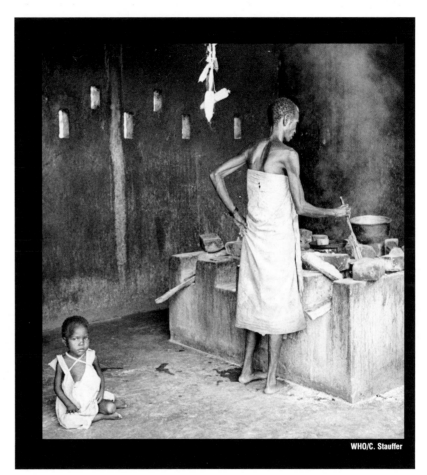

WHO/C. Stauffer

Cor pulmonale, an often fatal complication of chronic bronchitis, affects many women early in life. Early onset in women is thought to be due to domestic air pollution.

Proportion of men and women who collect water, by age, Kenya, 1983

Fetching water is the responsibility of women in most parts of the world. The health implications include skeletal damage, accidents, energy depletion and miscarriage.

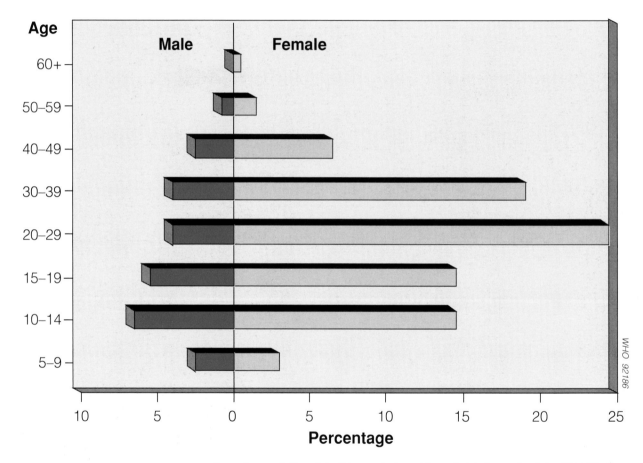

Source: Ferguson A. Women's health in a marginal area of Kenya. *Social science and medicine*, 1986, 23(1): 23.

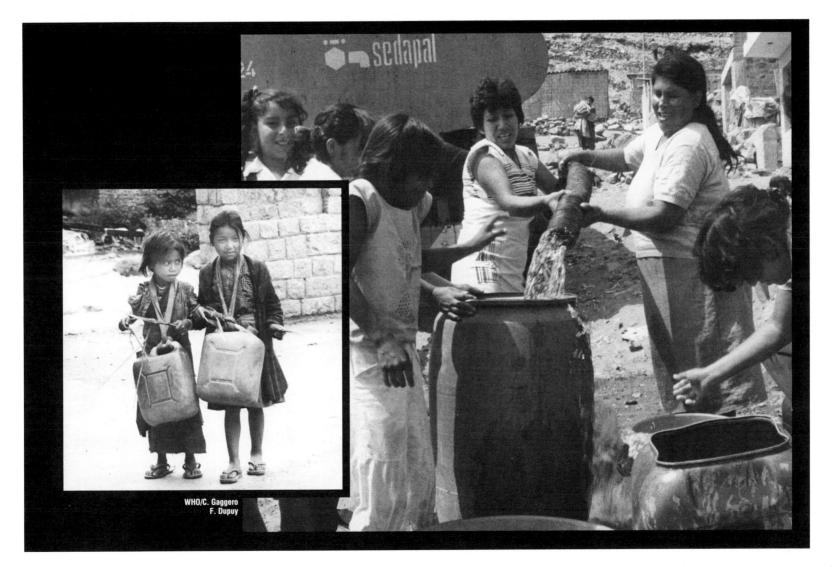

WHO/C. Gaggero
F. Dupuy

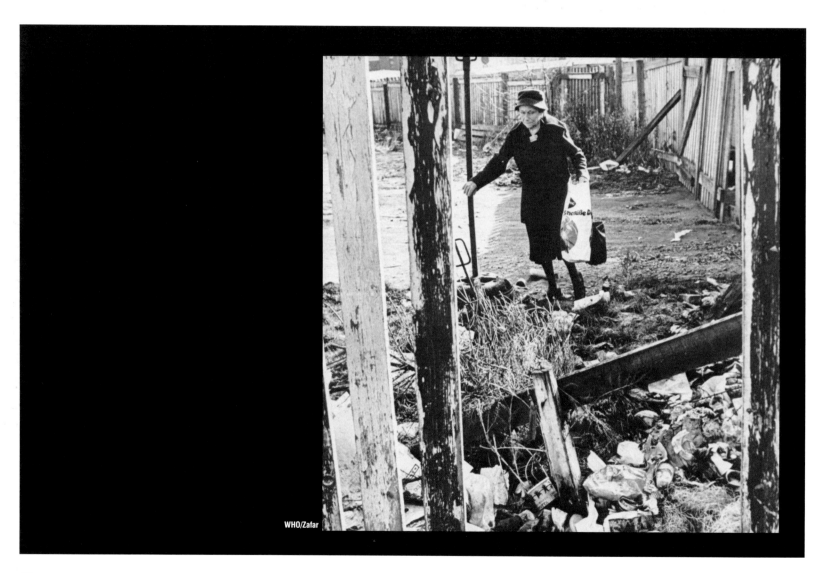

WHO/Zafar

Incidence of selected cancers in women in mining districts compared with those in non-mining districts of Czechoslovakia, 1985-86

Environmental pollution continues to have detrimental effects on populations. What are the special consequences for women?

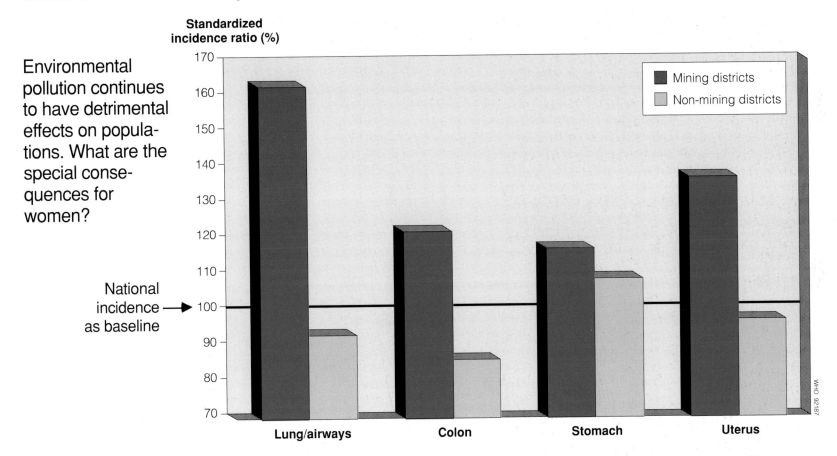

Source: Hertzman C. *Environment and health in Czechoslovakia.* Washington, DC, World Bank, 1990 (Internal report).

WHO 92187

Blood lead in children and mothers in various places within Katowice Region, Poland

Place	Children		Mothers	
	Mean blood level (μg/dl)	% with level >35 μg/dl	Mean blood level (μg/dl)	% with level >35 μg/dl
Szopienice	26.7	17.8	21.1	12.2
Miasteczko Sl	24.7	16.6	21.6	14.7
Zyglin	26.1	21.8	20.1	9.7
Lubowice*	12.7	0	10.6	0
Zabrze	18.9	3.2	15.9	3.5
Toszek	17.9	13.2	13.1	4.5
Bytom	15.2	10.0	15.5	5.1
Bojszow*	12.3	0	11.5	0
Brzeziny Sl	22.4	13.0	17.6	6.9
Brzozowice	23.4	7.8	16.8	4.8

* Relatively far from a source of contamination
15 μg/dl is the lowest adverse effect level. >25 μg/dl requires medical investigation.
Source: Centers for Disease Control, USA

Source: Hertzman C. *Poland: health and environment in the context of socioeconomic decline.* Washington, DC, World Bank, 1990 (Internal report).

Heavily contaminated soil is a significant source of exposure to lead for women and has been shown to cause neurological damage.

Pregnancy and childbirth

- Family planning and the quality of life

- Pregnancy and lactation as a percentage of women's reproductive years in selected countries

- Average number of children born per woman

- Estimated prevalence of nutritional anaemia in women

- Civil registration data: abortion deaths as a percentage of all maternal deaths

- Ratio of abortions to 1000 live births, all ages, around 1989 in Europe

- Effects of the introduction of an anti-abortion law in Romania in November 1966

- Estimates of maternal mortality: developed and developing countries

- Selected health indicators and their relationship to literacy, selected countries

- Characteristics of women with vesico-vaginal fistula

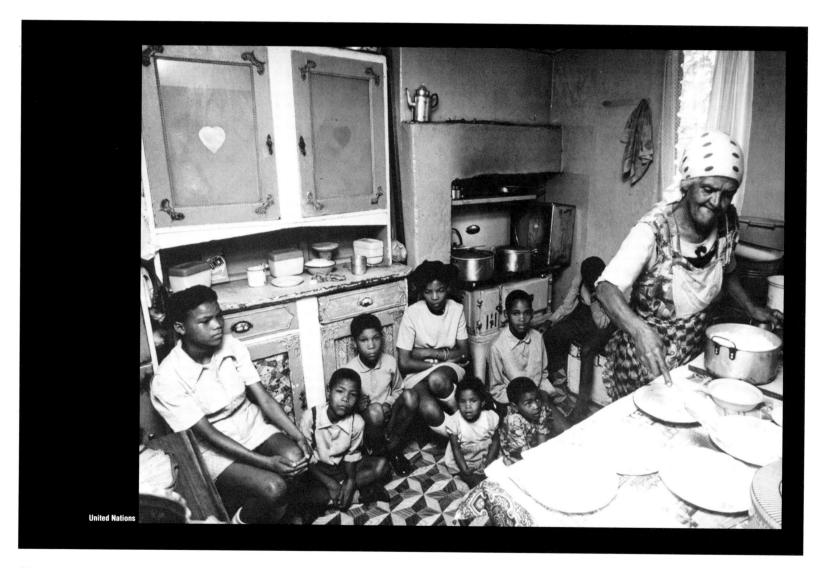

United Nations

Family planning and the quality of life

Issues of women's health were commonly equated with maternal health. Yet the "safety" of motherhood is now known to depend upon women's health from before birth through adult life, and upon a number of social and economic factors related to the status of women. It is no longer possible to consider maternal health in isolation from the broader spectrum of women, health and development.

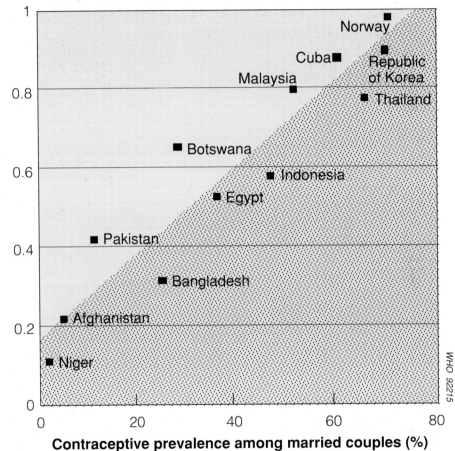

Human development index

Contraceptive prevalence among married couples (%)

WHO 92215

Source: Sadik N. T*he state of world population 1991.* New York, United Nations Population Fund, 1991, p. 17.

Pregnancy and lactation as a percentage of women's reproductive years in selected countries, around 1985

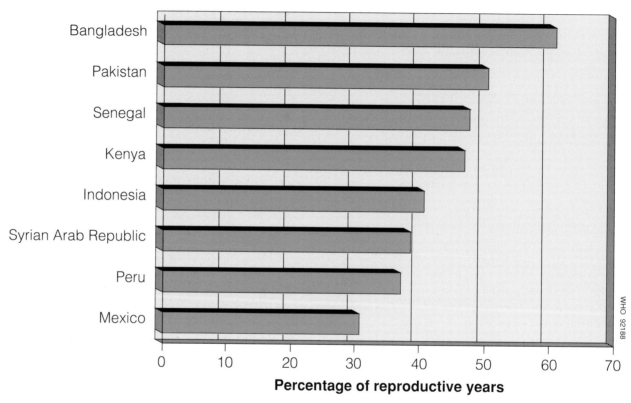

Percentage of reproductive years

Source: *Women, health and development.* Progress report by the Director-General. Report prepared for the 44th World Health Assembly. Geneva, World Health Organization, 1991 (unpublished document A44/15), p. 9.

In many countries, women spend close to half of their adult lives pregnant or lactating. The "maternal depletion syndrome" is well known, as is the enormity of the problem of nutritional anaemia, but how much do we understand of the implications for future generations? What are the dynamics of the interactions with the common diseases?

Average number of children born per woman

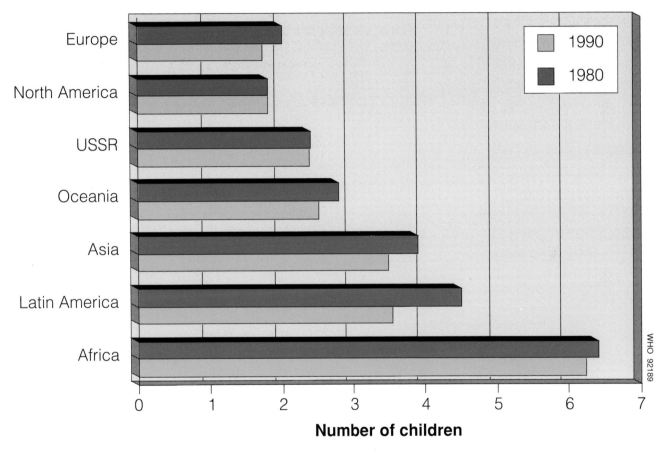

Number of children

Source: Based on data from *World population prospects 1990.* New York, United Nations, Department of International Economic and Social Affairs, 1991.

Estimated prevalence of nutritional anaemia in women, around 1990

An estimated 44% of women in developing countries suffer from nutritional anaemia, compared with 12% of women in developed countries. This is both a direct and indirect cause of maternal mortality. In addition it reduces work capacity, increases fatigue and increases susceptibility to health problems.

Region	Pregnant women	Non-pregnant women	All women
World	51%	35%	36%
Developing countries	55%	42%	44%
Developed countries	17%	12%	12%
Africa	51%	40%	42%
Asia	59%	44%	45%
Latin America	41%	30%	34%
North America	24%	10%	13%
Europe	17%	10%	10%

Source: *The prevalence of nutritional anaemia in women in the world.* Geneva, World Health Organization, 1992 (unpublished document WHO/MCH/MSM/92.2)

Civil registration data: abortion deaths as a percentage of all maternal deaths

Country	% maternal deaths
Romania, 1984	86
Chile, 1986	36
Argentina, 1985	35
Costa Rica, 1986	30
USSR, 1986	29
Paraguay (part), 1986	14
Sri Lanka, 1983	13
Peru, 1983	11
Mexico, 1983	10
Ecuador, 1986	9
France, 1986	8

Source: Royston E. Estimating the number of abortion deaths. In: Coeytaux F, Leonard A. Royston E, eds. *Methodological issues in abortion research.* New York, The Population Council, 1989, p. 24.

Ratio of abortions to 1000 live births, all ages, around 1989 in Europe

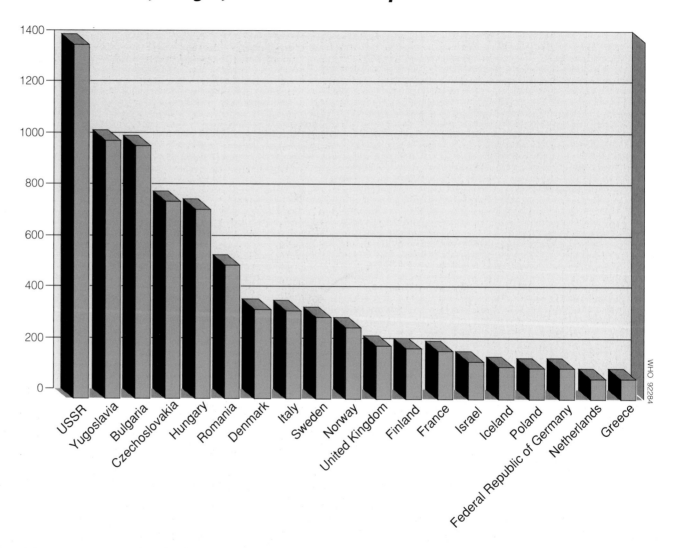

WHO 92284

Source: WHO, Regional Office for Europe. *Epidemiology, statistics and research*, Health for All database.

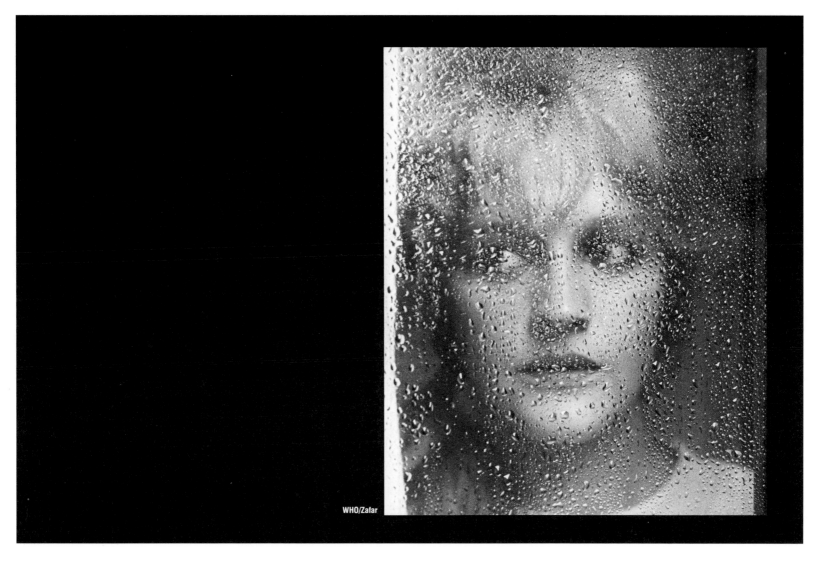

WHO/Zafar

Effects of the introduction of an anti-abortion law in Romania in November 1966

Birth rate/mortality rate

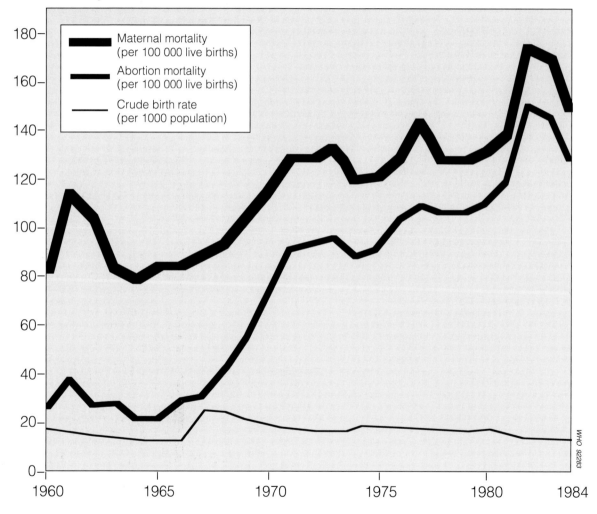

Source: Royston E, Armstrong S. *Preventing maternal deaths.* Geneva, World Health Organization, 1989, p. 116.

Estimates of maternal mortality: developed and developing countries, 1988

The huge discrepancy in maternal mortality between developed and developing countries amounts to a gap of neglect. A large proportion of maternal deaths could be prevented if women had access to care and information.

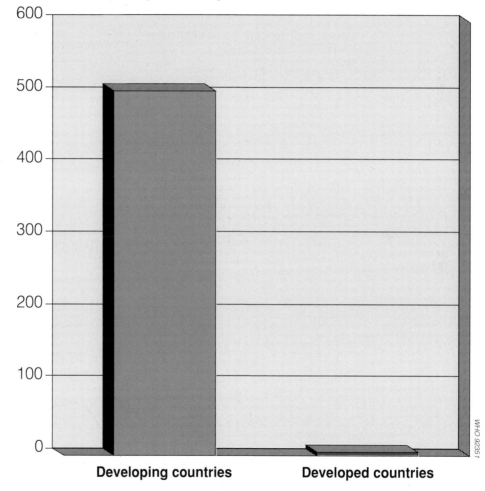

No. of maternal deaths (thousands)

Developing countries   Developed countries

WHO 92351

Source: New estimates of maternal mortality. *Weekly epidemiological record*, 1991, 66(47): 346

Selected health indicators and their relationship to literacy, selected countries

	Female adult literacy rate (%) (1990)[1]	Male adult literacy rate (%) (1990)[1]	Maternal mortality rate per 100 000 live births *[2]	Infant mortality rate per 1000 live births (1985-1990)[3]	% of births attended by trained personnel *[4]	% infants with low birth weight (< 2500g) (1991)[5]	Contraceptive prevalence rate among married women (%) (1980s)[6]
Nigeria	40	62	589 (1988) (Ibadan)	105	40 (1980)	16	5
Uganda	35	62	400-700 (1989)	103	38 (1988)	17	—
India	34	62	460 (1984)	99	30-35 (1985)	33	34
Morocco	38	61	327 (1978-80) (Casablanca)	82	20 (1979-80)	9	26
Zaire	61	84	200-800 (1980)	83	—	15	—
Egypt	34	63	500 (1981)	65	34 (1983-88)	104	30
Côte d'Ivoire	40	67	1800 (1988-89) (Abidjan)	96	20 (1987)	14	3
Zambia	65	80	105 (1983-88)	80	47 (1984) (Luampungo)	13	—
Indonesia	68	84	400 (1987)	75	36 (1982-87)	14	38
Italy	96	98	8 (1988)	11	100 (1982-87)	5.2	79

* National data except where indicated otherwise.

Sources: (1) Based on *Compendium of statistics on illiteracy*, Paris, UNESCO, 1990, No. 31.
(2) *Maternal mortality ratios and rates. A tabulation of available information, 3rd edition.* World Health Organization, Geneva, 1991 (unpublished document WHO/MCH/MSM/91.10).
(3) *UN World Population Prospects, 1990.*
(4) *Maternal mortality. A global factbook.* World Health Organization, Geneva, 1991 (unpublished document WHO/MCH/MSM/91.3).
(5) Division of Family Health. Database on low birthweight estimates, 27 March 1992.
(6) United Nations Population Division. *World contraceptives use*, 1987.

This table shows the relationship between women's literacy and several health indicators. How do social and economic factors affect access to obstetric care? Or availability of resources for improved maternal health and nutrition? What types of social control affect women's choices and access to services?

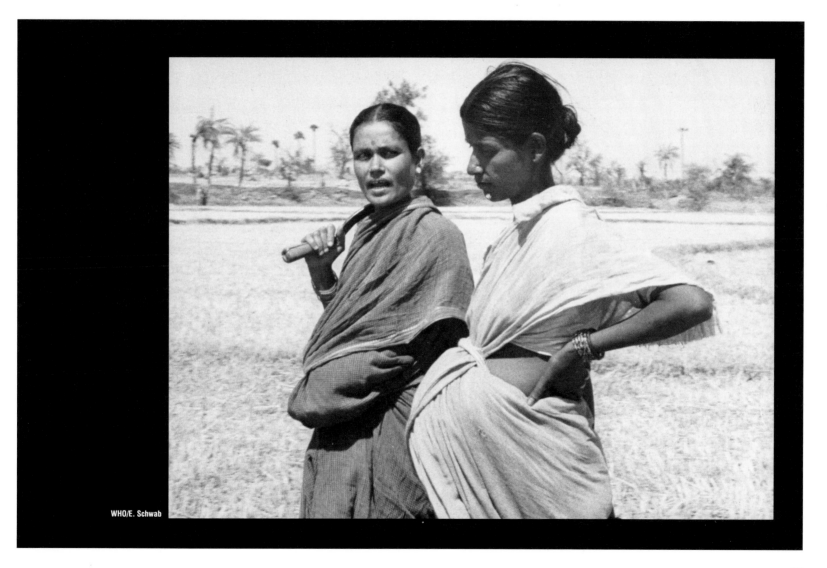

WHO/E. Schwab

Characteristics of women with vesico-vaginal fistula (VVF)

In Zaria, Nigeria, 77% of long-term fistula patients (those who had been incontinent for two years or more) were living apart from their husbands, while none of the control group was divorced or living apart.

Childlessness was found to be an important factor in marital breakdown. Of 174 fistula patients, 50 had living children before developing fistula. Of these 50, 14% were divorced as a result of the disorder, compared with 36% of the 124 patients with no living children.[1]

In India and Pakistan, as many as 80% or 90% of fistula patients are abandoned or divorced by their husbands.[2]

Someone who smells strongly of urine is not welcome in society. Women with fistulae usually become outcasts, not permitted to live in the same house as their families or husbands, not allowed to handle food, cook, or pray, not allowed to get on a bus. Some even have to leave their native village.[3]

It is often said that maternal mortality is only the tip of the iceberg; estimates of morbidity associated with childbearing run into the millions. Obstetric fistulae, including vesico-vaginal fistula, are an example of a widespread problem with serious health and social consequences.

Sources: [1] Murphy M. Social consequences of vesico-vaginal fistula in northern Nigeria. *Journal of biosocial sciences*, 1981, 13:139-150.

[2] Buckshee K, New Delhi, personal communication, 1989 and Hanif H, Lahore, Pakistan, personal communication, 1989.

[3] Dali SM, Kathmandu, Nepal, personal communication, 1989.

All cited in: *Obstetric fistulae. A review of available information:* Geneva, World Health Organization, 1991 (unpublished document WHO/MCH/MSM/91.5), p.7.

Diseases and infections

- Prevalence of reproductive tract infections (RTIs) among selected female populations in developing countries

- The annual total of sexually transmitted infections

- Prevalence of gonorrhoea in studies of pregnant women

- Percentage of pregnant women with bacteriological evidence of C. trachomatis in specific studies

- Number of infertile women as a percentage of all women

- Estimated/projected annual HIV infections, by sex

- Cumulative global HIV/AIDS estimates

- Number of HIV-infected African women and number of infected/uninfected children born to them

- Mortality rates for women aged 20 to 35 years in New York City

- Distribution of patients positive for malaria attending clinics in Maesot district, Thailand

- Distribution of males and females testing positive for malaria at community level

- Estimated distribution of deaths from various smoking-related diseases among women in developed countries

- Most frequent cancers in women, by region, with estimated annual number of cases in thousands

- Percentages of three most frequent cancers in women, developed and developing countries

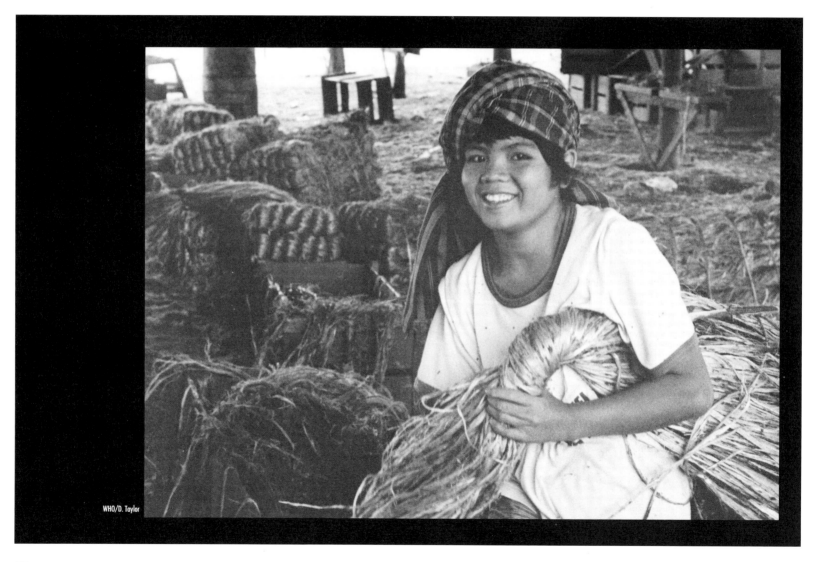

WHO/D. Taylor

The interactions between women's status and diseases need more attention. We have an incomplete understanding of:

■ *gender differences in prevalence:*
do health statistics accurately reflect the numbers of women with malaria? tuberculosis? if women have less access to services, are they included in the statistics? are women invisible to health statisticians?

■ *gender differences in utilization of services for prevention or control:*
are women less likely to come for treatment? are health education campaigns relevant to women? are service schedules suited to women's working day?

■ *the effects of diseases/infections during pregnancy and lactation:*
much is known about malaria during pregnancy and the transmission of sexually transmitted diseases from mother to baby, but are there sufficient data on tuberculosis during pregnancy?

■ *the social implications for women:*
men and women experience very different consequences of diseases – what social stigma is suffered by women with leprosy? with guinea worm infection? what happens to a woman's marriage if she has filariasis? what are the economic consequences for women with malaria as compared with men? what happens to women's roles as carers in the family?

Prevalence of reproductive tract infections (RTIs) among selected female populations* in developing countries

Reproductive tract infections (RTIs) have been hidden in the "culture of silence". They are known to all women in the world; when left untreated, they represent a vast reservoir of infection with serious short-term and long-term effects on women's overall health status. RTIs have an impact on a range of issues, including maternal functions, sexually transmitted diseases, HIV/AIDS, fatigue, and child survival.

Infection	Africa	Asia	Latin America
Gonorrhoea			
Prevalence	40%	0.3-12%	2-18%
Number of studies	39	9	5
Chlamydia			
Prevalence	4-23%	2-14%	
Number of studies	5	2	
Trichomoniasis			
Prevalence	2-50%	5-30%	3-24%
Number of studies	15	4	5

* Populations include family planning clients, gynaecology clients, prenatal clinic patients, women giving birth in clinical settings, and community-based populations. Studies on female populations presenting specifically with pelvic inflammatory disease or puerperal sepsis have been excluded from this summary as have clients of sexually transmitted disease clinics.

Source: Wasserheit J. Significance and scope of reproductive tract infections among Third World women. *International journal of gynaecology and obstetrics*, 1989, suppl. 3: 154.

Dixon-Mueller R, Wasserheit J. *The culture of silence. Reproductive tract infections among women in the Third World.* New York, International Women's Health Coalition, 1991.

Sexually transmitted diseases are the most commonly reported infectious diseases, and are increasing. Gender differences in transmission, symptoms and treatment may not be adequately understood or appreciated by health authorities. To what extent is the double sexual standard taken into account when approaches to health services or information programmes are being developed?

The annual total of sexually transmitted infections, 1990

Disease	No. of cases
Trichomoniasis	120 million
Genital chlamydia	50 million
Genital papillomavirus	30 million
Gonorrhoea	25 million
Genital herpes	20 million
HIV infection	1 million
Syphilis	3.5 million
Chancroid	2 million

Percentage of pregnant women with bacteriological evidence of C. trachomatis in specific studies

Country	Percentage positive
Fiji	45.1
Gabon	9.9
Gambia	6.9
Ghana	7.7
Kenya	29.0
Nigeria	6.5
Somalia	18.8
Thailand	12.8

Prevalence of gonorrhoea in studies of pregnant women

Country	Prevalence (%)
Cameroon	15.0
Central African Republic	9.5
Fiji	2.3
Gambia	6.7
Gabon	5.5
Ghana	4.4
Jamaica	11.0
Kenya	6.6
Malaysia	0.5
Nigeria	5.2
Senegal	2.1
Singapore	0.8
South Africa	11.7
Swaziland	3.9
Thailand	11.9
Uganda	40
United Republic of Tanzania	6.0
Zambia	11.3
Zimbabwe	7.0

Source: De Schryver A, Meheus A. Epidemiology of sexually transmitted diseases: the global picture. *Bulletin of the World Health Organization*, 1990, 68(5): 639-654.

Number of infertile women as a percentage of all women*

One of the effects of reproductive tract infections and sexually transmitted diseases is infertility, which represents a personal tragedy for families in all settings, and is an important public health concern in a number of countries. Are the consequences the same for men and women? What happens to childless women?

	date	primary infertility (%)	secondary infertility (%)
Benin	1988	3	10
Brazil	1988	2	30
Cameroon	1988	12	33
Gabon	1987	32	
Mozambique	1987	14	
Pakistan	1988	4	24
Senegal	1978	6	13
United Republic of Tanzania (urban)	1986	5	20
(rural)	1986	4	19

*In some instances surveys were restricted to married women.

Source: Abstracted from *Infertility: A tabulation of available data on prevalence of primary and secondary infertility.* Geneva, World Health Organization, 1991 (unpublished document WHO/MCH/91.9).

It is known that the development of leprosy is accelerated during pregnancy. What other mechanisms are at work? The social consequences of leprosy are vastly different for women and men. Often women are outcasts; their marriages end.

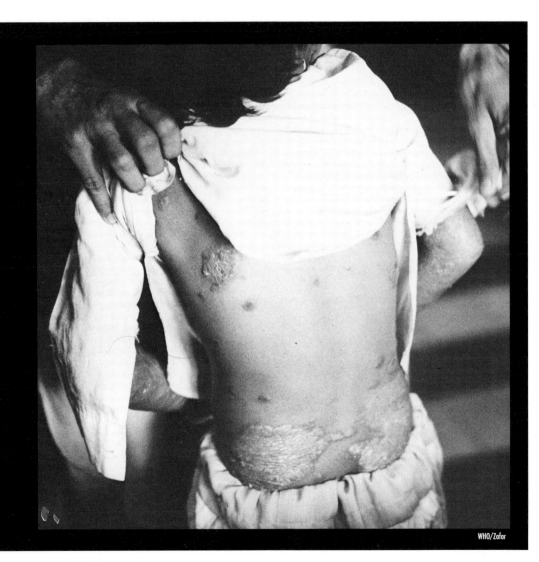

WHO/Zafar

The rise in HIV infection and AIDS in women has become a great concern of the 1990s. Initially, the importance of heterosexual transmission and transmission to the fetus was not fully appreciated. An understanding of the interrelationship between women's status and HIV/AIDS is critical to the future spread of the disease. How can women gain control to prevent transmission? Can they insist that their partners use a condom? How can information best reach women? What kinds of changes can work fast enough to help women with few choices? What types of interventions can help women cope with their own illness, that of their husbands or their children, and with others suffering from the disease? Are women the main care-givers?

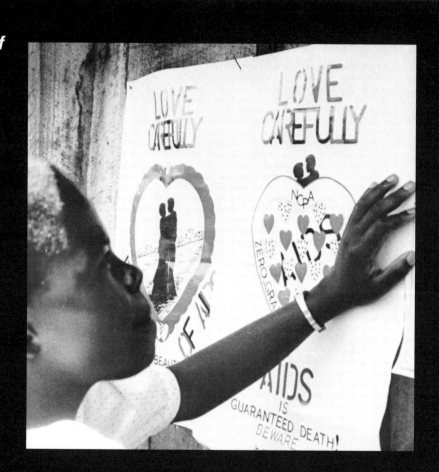

WHO/J.&.P. Hubley

Estimated/projected annual HIV infections, by sex

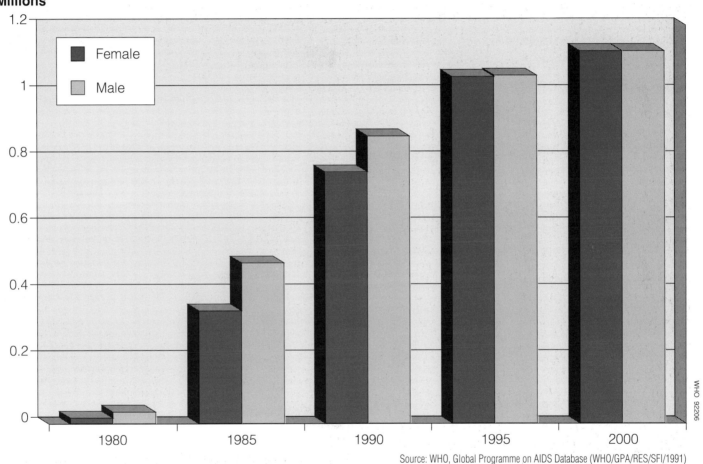

Millions

Source: WHO, Global Programme on AIDS Database (WHO/GPA/RES/SFI/1991)

WHO 92206

These projections show little difference in the adult infection rates in men and women by the mid-1990s.

Cumulative global HIV/AIDS estimates, January 1992

Millions of children will die of AIDS in the next decade. Do women have any choices that can prevent the death of their children? Who will be blamed for the deaths of so many children? Can future generations ever forgive us?

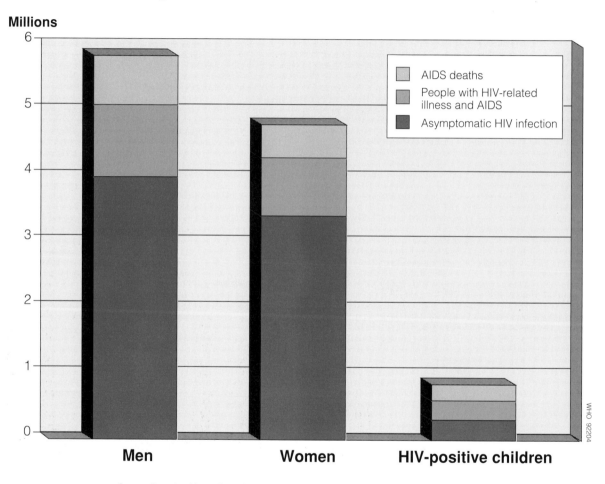

Source: *Current and future dimensions of the HIV/AIDS pandemic: a capsule summary.* Geneva, World Health Organization, 1992 (unpublished document WHO/GPA/RES/SFI/92.1).

Number of HIV-infected African women and number of infected/uninfected children born to them

Millions

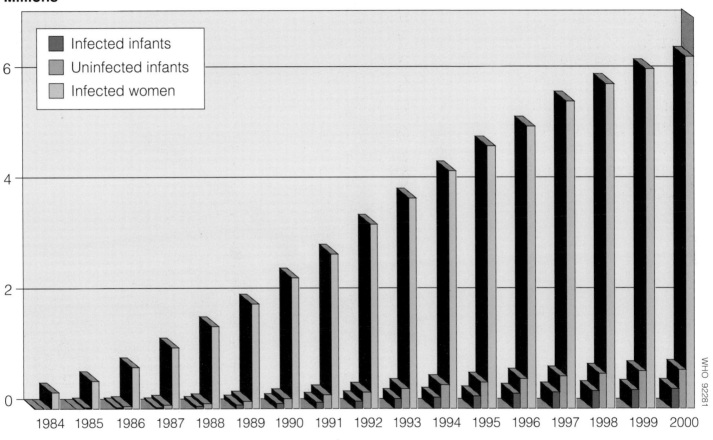

Legend:
- Infected infants
- Uninfected infants
- Infected women

Source: WHO, Global Programme on AIDS Database (WHO/GPA/RES/SFI)

WHO 92281

The number of children infected is likely to increase. What have we yet to learn about children with AIDS? About women's reproduction and AIDS?

Mortality rates for women aged 20 to 35 years in New York City

Mortality rate per 100 000 women

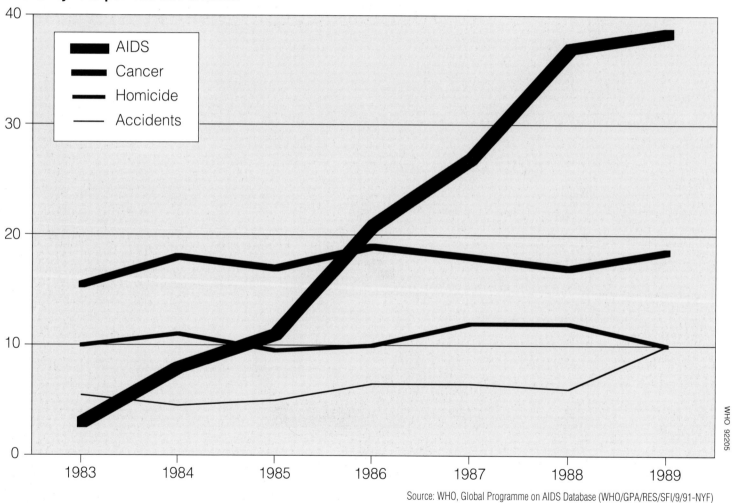

Source: WHO, Global Programme on AIDS Database (WHO/GPA/RES/SFI/9/91-NYF)

WHO 92205

While tuberculosis is declining rapidly in the industrialized world, it is showing little decrease in the majority of developing countries. Globally, 1700 million people are infected, and more than 20 million of them have active tuberculosis. Some 80% of cases in the developing world occur in the most productive age group (15-59 years), where the disease accounts for more than a quarter of avoidable deaths. What are the implications for women?

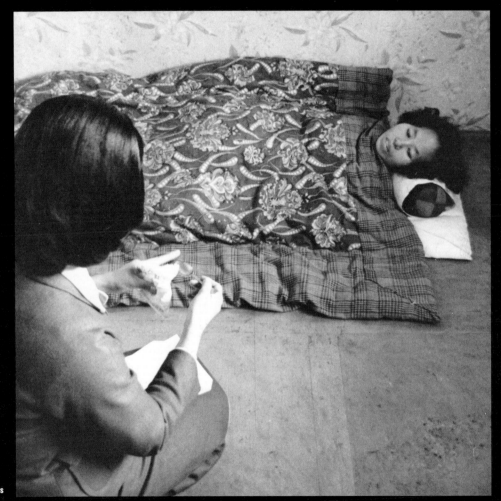

WHO/P. Boucas

Distribution of patients positive for malaria attending clinics in Maesot district, Thailand, 1985–1986

Age (years)	Sex	Maesot clinic	Popphra clinic	Mobile clinic	Sub-totals
0 - 15	M	87 (2%)	124 (19%)	207 (33%)	418 (7%)
	F	46 (1%)	86 (13%)	156 (25%)	288 (5%)
16 - 30	M	2936 (62%)	243 (37%)	155 (25%)	3334 (56%)
	F	458 (10%)	79 (12%)	37 (6%)	574 (10%)
31- 45	M	741 (16%)	68 (11%)	51 (8%)	860 (14%)
	F	93 (2%)	20 (3%)	9 (1%)	122 (2%)
>45	M	290 (6%)	20 (3%)	9 (1%)	319 (5%)
	F	70 (1%)	11 (2%)	8 (1%)	89 (1%)
Total		4721(100%)	651(100%)	632(100%)	6004(100%)

Distribution of males (●) and females (▲) testing positive for malaria at community level

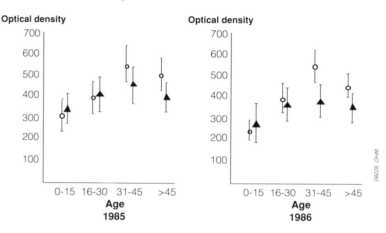

Mean positive optical densities in enzyme-linked immunosorbent assay, with 95% confidence limits in Maesot District, Thailand, 1985 and 1986, for males (●) and females (▲) of different age groups

Source: Ettling M et al. Evaluation of malaria clinics in Maesot, Thailand: use of serology to assess coverage. *Transactions of the Royal Society of Tropical Medicine and Hygiene*, 1989, 83: 328.

The table and graphs above show that the proportion of women testing positive for malaria is greater at the community level than in the clinics. Seroepidemiological findings from a random sample of over 500 villagers in the area show similar exposure rates among men and women of similar age. By contrast, the figures show a predominance of young men among patients treated in the Maesot clinics (56% of all cases).

How accurate are malaria prevalence figures based on health service data? Are health authorities leaving women out of their calculations? Why are women not coming to health services for treatment of malarial symptoms? What does this mean for malaria control strategies?

Estimated distribution of deaths from various smoking-related diseases among women in developed countries, 1985

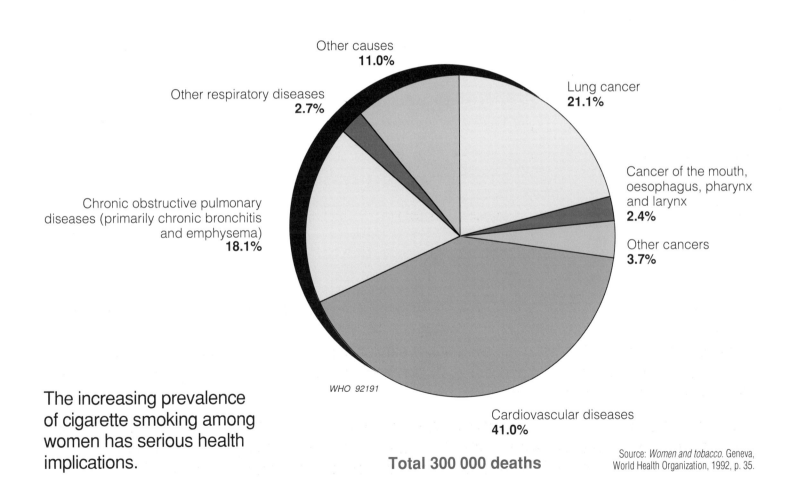

Other causes
11.0%

Other respiratory diseases
2.7%

Lung cancer
21.1%

Chronic obstructive pulmonary diseases (primarily chronic bronchitis and emphysema)
18.1%

Cancer of the mouth, oesophagus, pharynx and larynx
2.4%

Other cancers
3.7%

WHO 92191

Cardiovascular diseases
41.0%

The increasing prevalence of cigarette smoking among women has serious health implications.

Total 300 000 deaths

Source: *Women and tobacco.* Geneva, World Health Organization, 1992, p. 35.

Most frequent cancers in women, by region, with estimated annual number of cases in thousands, late 1970s

Region	Most common	Second most common	Third most common
North America	Breast (105)	Colorectal (56)	Lung (25)
Latin America	Breast (49)	Cervix (44)	Stomach (17)
Europe	Breast (162)	Colorectal (87)	Stomach (61)
USSR	Stomach (49)	Cervix (31)	Breast (31)
Africa	Cervix (37)	Breast (27)	Lymphatic (12)
Australia/New Zealand	Breast (6)	Colorectal (4)	Cervix (1)
Japan	Stomach (29)	Breast (12)	Cervix (10)
China	Cervix (132)	Stomach (68)	Oesophagus (59)
India and other Asia	Cervix (142)	Breast (95)	Mouth* (48)

* Mouth and pharynx

Source: Stanley K, Stjernsward J, Koraltchouk V. Women and cancer. *World health statistics quarterly*, 1987, 40(3): 268.

Percentages of three most frequent cancers in women, developed and developing countries, late 1970s

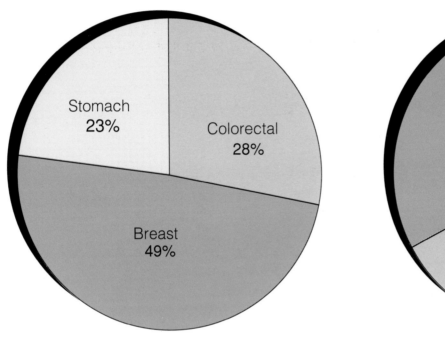

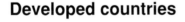

Developed countries

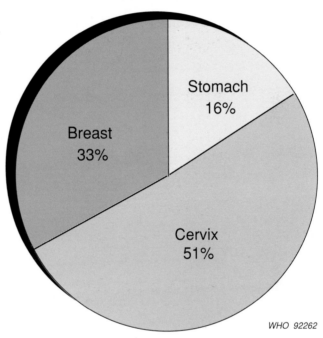

WHO 92262

Developing countries

Source: data from Stanley K, Stjernsward J, Koraltchouk V. Women and cancer.
World health statistics quarterly, 1987, 40(3): 268.

The differences in cancer frequencies between developed and developing countries are most striking with regard to cervical cancer. What strategies can be devised for the diagnosis and treatment of cervical cancer in developing countries? What actions are needed to limit cancer deaths among women?

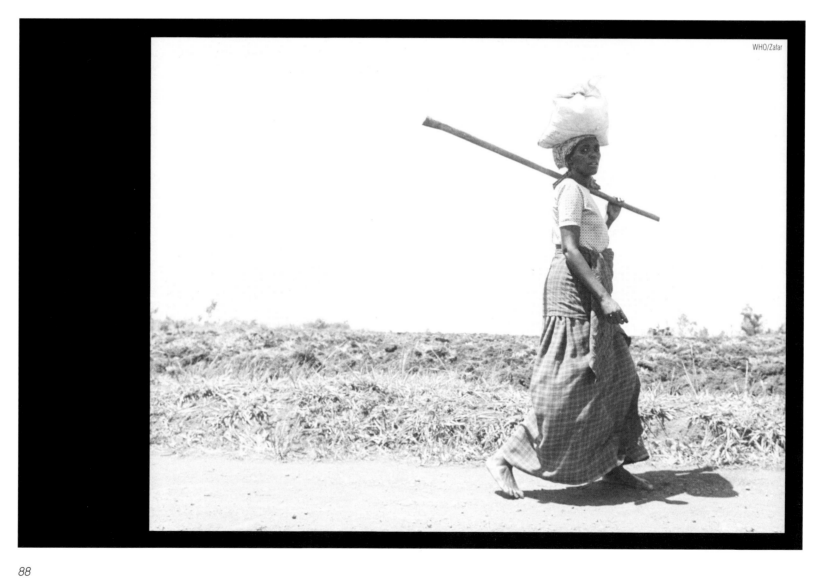

WHO/Zafar

Violence and mental disorders

- Reported types of violence against women

- Annual incidence of specific mental disorders per 100 person-years of risk by sex and age

- Lifetime prevalence of any mental disorder, and percentage receiving treatment

"In Norway, 25% of female gynaecology patients have been physically or sexually abused by their mates."

"In Bangkok, a study showed that 50% of married women are beaten regularly by their husbands."

"In Kenya, in a detailed family planning survey, it was found that 42% of women said they were beaten regularly by their husbands."

"In Peru, 70% of all crimes reported to police are of women beaten by their husbands."

"In Papua New Guinea, 67% of rural, and 56% of urban women were victims of wife abuse."

"A study of causes of female mortality in Bangladesh showed 12.3% female mortality due to intentional injury."

Source: Heise L. Violence against women: the missing agenda. In: Koblinsky M, Gay J, Timyan J, eds. *The health of women: a global perspective.* Boulder, CO, Westview Press, forthcoming publication, p. 169, p. 179.

"In Santiago, a survey showed that 80% of women have suffered physical, emotional or sexual abuse by a male partner or relative."[1]

"In Colombia, a national survey showed that 65% of women declared that they had been hit by their husband or companion."[2]

"In India in 1990, police officially recorded 4,835 dowry deaths in all of India, but the Ahmedabad Women's Action group estimates that 1000 women have been burned alive annually in Gujarat State alone."[1]

"In the USA, every 15 seconds, a woman is beaten, and four battered women die each day."[1]

"In Caracas, Venezuela, in the first week after establishment of the Municipal Service for Women in 1985, 89% of the cases dealt with charges of severe physical abuse of women by their partners."[3]

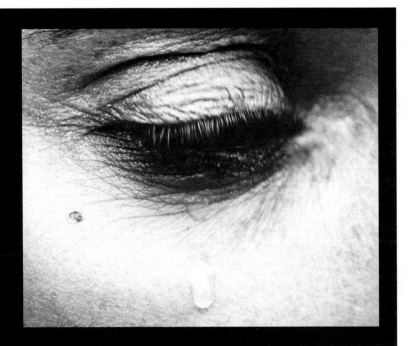

"The Forensic Clinic in La Paz, Bolivia, reported a total of 1,432 cases of physical assault during 1986, of which 954 (66%) involved women. Of these 954 cases, 60.7% were assaults by the woman's conjugal partner, 22.6% were rapes, and 16.7% were assaults by other family members or neighbours."[3]

Sources: (1) Heise L. Violence against women: the missing agenda. In: Koblinsky M, Gay J, Timyan J, eds. *The health of women: a global perspective.* Boulder, CO, Westview Press, forthcoming publication, p. 169.
(2) Profamilia. *Encuesta de prevalencia, demografia y salud 1990.* Bogota, Profamilia, 1991.
(3) *Epidemiological profile of women's health in the Region of the Americas.* Washington, DC, Pan American Health Organization, 1990 (unpublished document PAHO/PWD), p. 69.

Reported types of violence against women, mid 1980s

It is no longer possible for society to tolerate violence against women. The violence is hidden behind the doors of family homes in all countries across all boundaries – in rich and poor homes, in developed and developing countries. The emergency rooms of hospitals all over the world see beaten women; health workers in all services see the physical and mental damage that has been done. Can health authorities stay mute? Can they shrug off their responsibilities and "leave it to the police"?

Evidence from studies reveals that sexual abuse is "learned", and is passed on from one generation to another. How can health education programmes help to stop the vicious cycle? How can mental health programmes deal with the perpetrators and victims of such crimes?

Source: *The world's women 1970-1990. Trends and statistics.* New York, United Nations, 1991 (Social Statistics and Indicators, Series K, No. 8), p. 19.

	Domestic violence	Incest	Homicide in family	Sexual assault and rape	Sexual harassment
Developed regions					
Australia	X		X		
Austria	X		X		
Belgium	X	X		X	X
Canada	X		X	X	X
Finland	X	X		X	X
France				X	
Germany	X	X	X		X
Greece	X		X	X	
Italy		X		X	
New Zealand	X		X		
Poland	X				
Portugal				X	
Spain					X
United Kingdom	X			X	X
United States	X	X	X	X	X
Africa					
Kenya	X		X		
Nigeria	X				
Uganda	X				
Latin America and Caribbean					
Argentina	X				
Brazil	X			X	
Chile	X	X	X		
Colombia	X	X		X	
Dominican Republic			X		
Ecuador	X				
Jamaica	X	X		X	
Peru	X				
Puerto Rico			X		
Trinidad and Tobago	X	X		X	
Venezuela				X	
Asia and Pacific					
Bangladesh	X		X		
China			X		
India	X		X	X	X
Israel	X				
Kuwait	X				
Malaysia	X			X	
Philippines				X	
Thailand	X		X		

"In a Trinidad and Tobago study, female admissions for alcoholism increased between 1970 and 1980 from 2.4% to 10.0% of all female admissions, while admissions for women with drug dependence increased by 300% between 1970 and 1984."

"Sri Lanka suicide rates in women aged 15-24 are five times the rate of infectious diseases and 55 times that of obstetric related deaths."

Source: Paltiel F. Women's mental health: a global perspective. In: Koblinsky M, Gay J, Timyan J, eds. *The health of women. a global perspective.* Boulder, CO, Westview Press, forthcoming publication, p. 202, p. 170.

Psychiatric and psychological theories and methods have been based on male perceptions, and many of the existing ideas on women and mental health are therefore misleading. New approaches are now being developed based on social realities, bringing in women's experiences and voices.

Source: Dennerstein L, Astbury J, Morse C. *Psychosocial and mental health aspects of women's health.* Geneva, World Health Organization, 1992 (unpublished document, WHO/FHE).

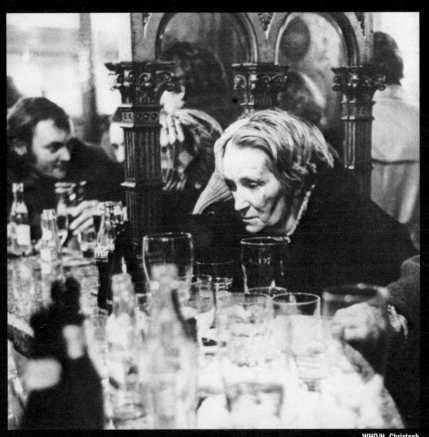

WHO/H. Christoph

Annual incidence of specific mental disorders per 100 person-years of risk by sex

Reviews of the prevalence of mental disorders conclude that, overall, rates among men and women are similar; however, as illustrated in the table, the nature of the disorders tends to be different.

Disorders	Male	Female	Total
Major depressive disorders	1.10	1.98	1.59
Panic disorders	0.30	0.76	0.56
Phobic disorders	2.33	5.38	3.98
Obsessive-compulsive disorders	0.39	0.92	0.69
Drug abuse/dependence	1.66	0.66	1.09
Alcohol abuse/dependence	3.67	0.61	1.79
Total	9.45	10.31	9.70

Source: Eaton WW et al. The incidence of specific DIS/DSM-III mental disorders: data from the NIMH epidemic catchment area programme, *Acta psychiatrica Scandinavica*, 1989, 79: 164.

Lifetime prevalence of any mental disorder, and percentage receiving treatment
NIMH/ECA* data (New Haven, Baltimore, St Louis)

The ECA study involved about 17 000 community residents in three sites. Distinct differences in the treatment of women and men were found. Furthermore, studies in the United Kingdom and the United States show that most women are treated by general practitioners while men receive specialized treatment.

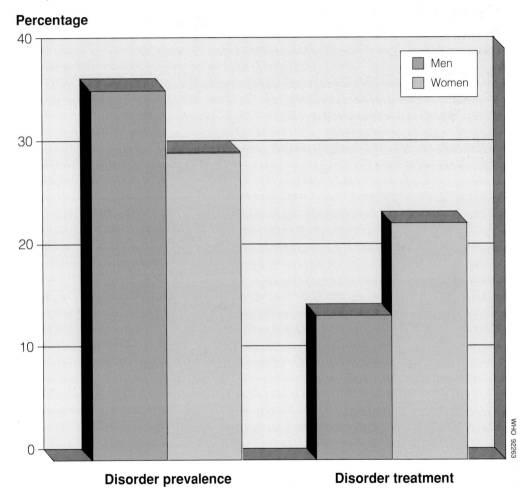

Percentage

Men
Women

Disorder prevalence   Disorder treatment

WHO 92263

*National Institute of Mental Health (NIMH)
Epidemiological Catchment Area Program (ECA)

Source: Paltiel F. Women's mental health: a global perspective. In: Koblinsky M, Gay J, Timyan J, eds. *The health of women. a global perspective.* Boulder, CO, Westview Press, forthcoming publication, p. 197.

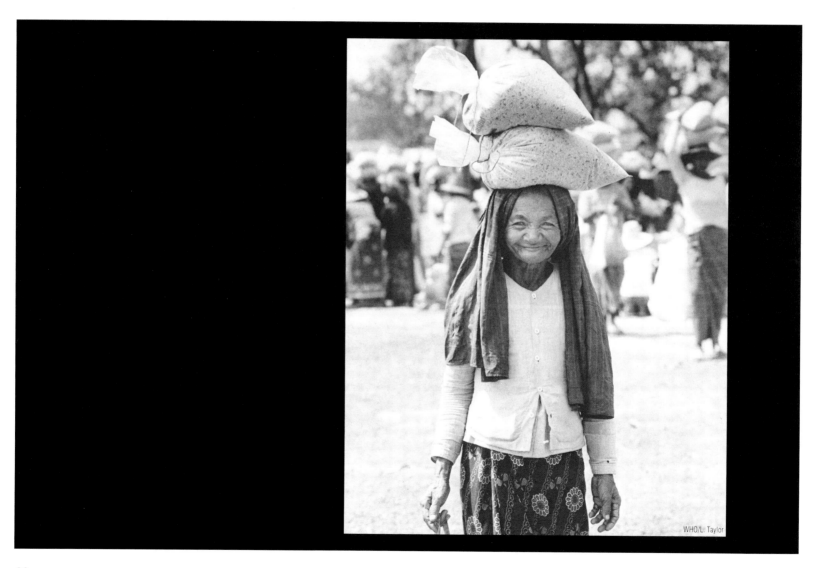

WHO/L. Taylor

Elderly women

- Life expectancy and disability-free life expectancy at birth, USA and England and Wales

- Population aged 65 and over in developed and developing countries by sex

- Percentage increase in number of widows aged 65 and over

- Percentage of specific age and sex groups living in rural areas

- Percentage of male population in urban areas, by age

- Crude death rates from cardiovascular diseases, by age and sex

- Age- and sex-specific distribution of generalized osteoarthritis (3 or more joints involved) in Indonesia

- Prevalence rate of definite rheumatoid arthritis in the USA and Indonesia among men and women aged 55 years and over

Life expectancy and disability-free life expectancy at birth

USA (1970 and 1980) and England and Wales (1976 and 1985)

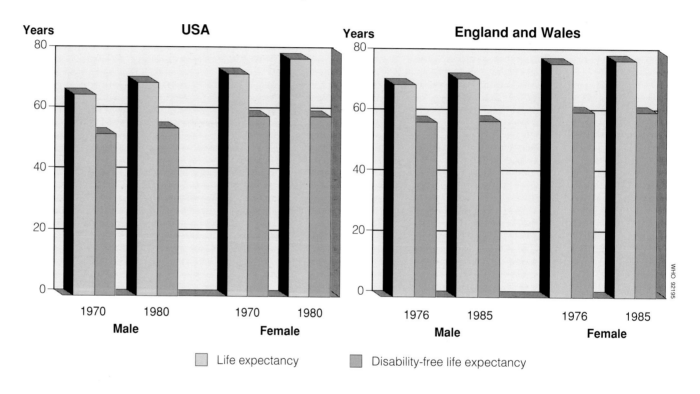

Source: *A paradigm for health: a framework for new public health action* - Discussion paper by the Director-General. Geneva, World Health Organization, 1992 (unpublished document EB89/11).

This graph shows that, while life expectancy is increasing, the number of years free from disability is stagnating. This phenomenon of living longer but not necessarily enjoying a good quality of life has implications for health services and family care, especially for women, who constitute the majority of elderly people.

Population aged 65 and over in developed and developing countries by sex, from 1970 to 2000

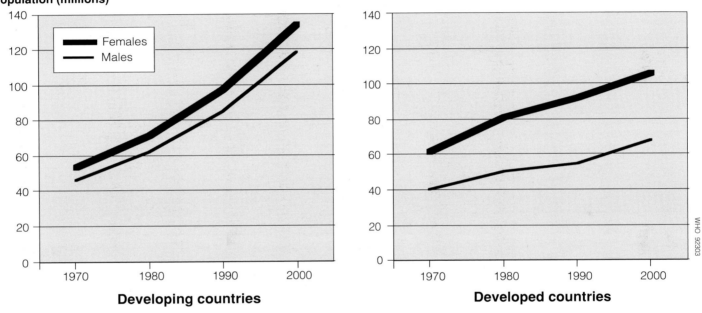

Population (millions)

Legend:
- Females
- Males

Developing countries

Developed countries

Source: *The sex and age distribution of population, 1990 revision.* New York, United Nations, 1990.

The increasing proportions of elderly people in the populations of both developed and developing countries indicate the need for greater attention to be paid to this group, most of whom are women.

Percentage increase in number of widows aged 65 and over

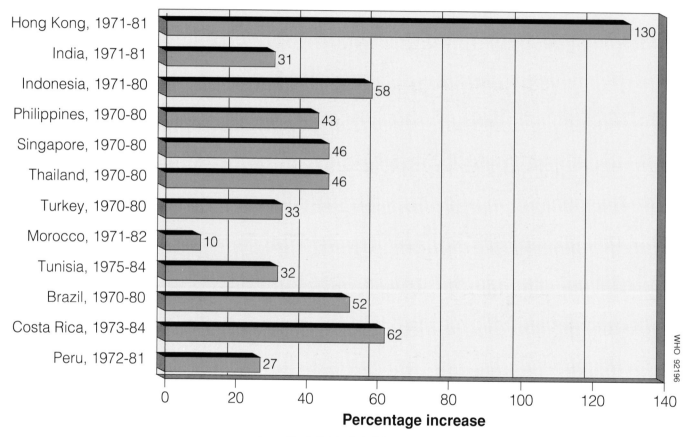

Source: Kinsella K. Aging in the Third World. In: Chaney EM, ed. *Empowering older women: cross-cultural views.*
Washington, DC, American Association of Retired Persons, 1990, p. 66

The percentage increase in the number of elderly widows is substantial.
What is happening to elderly women living alone? What is the effect of
increased migration and family dissolution on care of the elderly?

Percentage of population in rural areas by age and sex

Percentage of male population in urban areas, by age

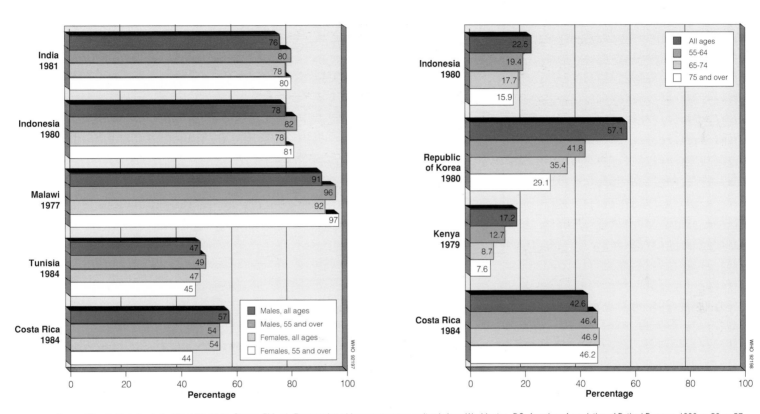

Source: Kinsella K. Aging in the Third World. In: Chaney EM, ed. *Empowering older women: cross-cultural views.* Washington, DC, American Association of Retired Persons, 1990, p. 56, p. 57.

As a result of the migration of young people to urban areas and, in some cases, the return of older people from urban areas to their rural homes, the rural population in most countries has a disproportionate number of elderly persons. What does this mean in terms of health care needs? What social safety networks are required? What type of infrastructure is needed to meet the daily life requirements of the elderly, such as accessibility to food, water and communications?

Crude death rates from cardiovascular diseases, by age and sex

The importance of cardiovascular diseases for women is shown here. A large study of women and men hospitalized for coronary heart disease in the USA in 1987 found that the women underwent fewer major diagnostic and therapeutic procedures than the men.

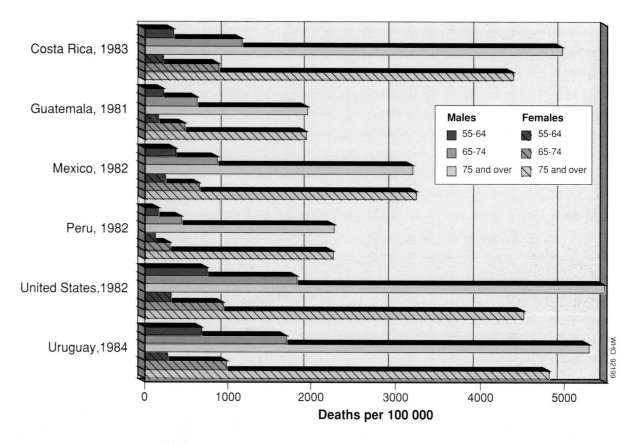

WHO 92199

Source: Kinsella K. Aging in the Third World. In: Chaney EM, ed. *Empowering older women: cross-cultural views.* Washington, DC, American Association of Retired Persons, 1990, p. 61.

Ayanian J, Epstein A. Differences in the use of procedures between women and men hospitalized for coronary heart disease. *New England journal of medicine*, 1991, 355(4): 221.

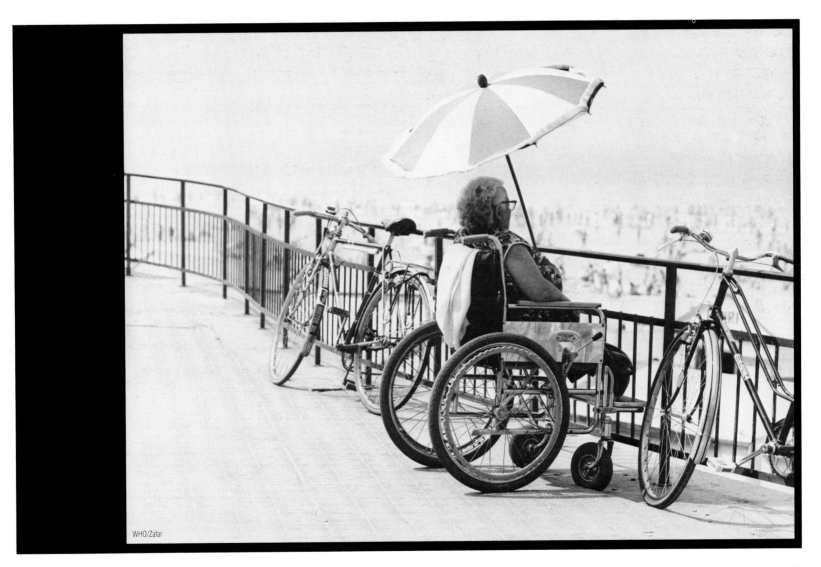

WHO/Zafar

Age- and sex-specific distribution of generalized osteoarthritis (3 or more joints involved) in Indonesia, early 1980s

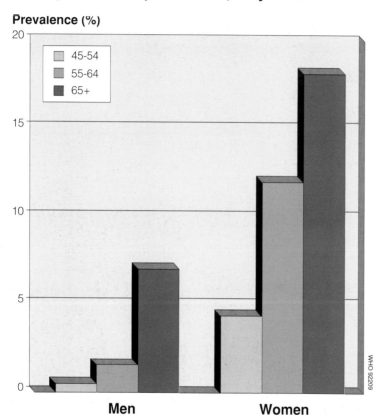

Prevalence rate of definite rheumatoid arthritis in the USA and Indonesia among men and women aged 55 years and over, early 1980s

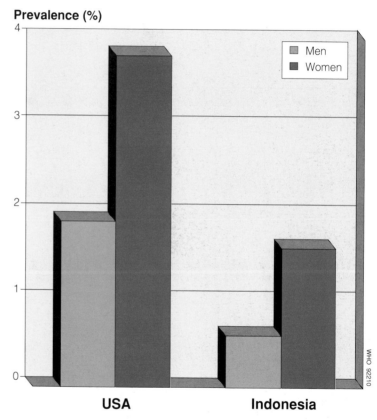

Source: based on data in Darmawan J. *Rheumatic conditions in the northern part of central Java: an epidemiological survey.* West Kalimantan, Geboren te Pontianak, 1988.

Osteoporosis is increasingly recognized as an important problem for elderly women. It is of particular concern that the elderly have multiple chronic disabilities.

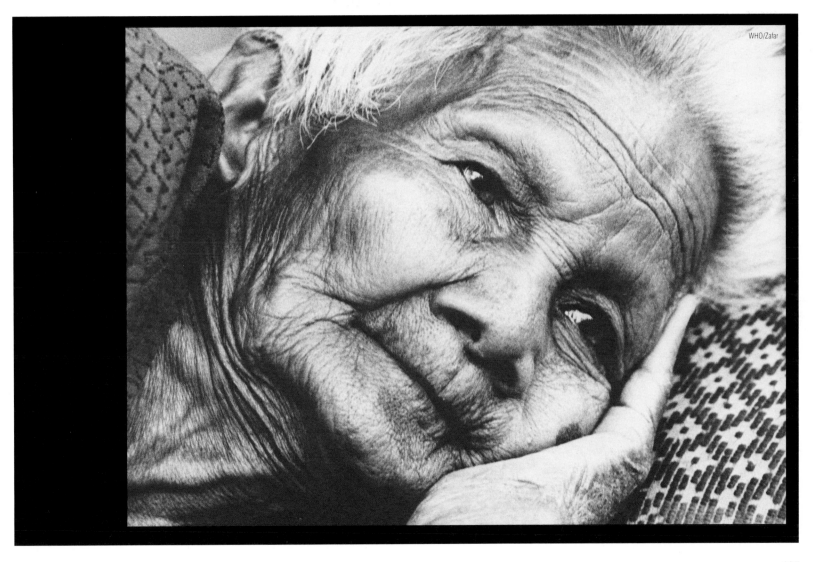

WHO/Zafar

Selected bibliography

AbouZahr C, Royston E. *Maternal mortality. A global factbook.* Geneva, World Health Organization, 1991 (unpublished document WHO/MCH/MSM/91.3).[1]

Ayanian J, Epstein A. Differences in the use of procedures between women and men hospitalized for coronary heart disease. *New England journal of medicine*, 1991, 355(4):221-225.

Bown L. *Preparing the future - women, literacy and development.* Chard, Somerset, ActionAid, undated (ActionAid Development Report No. 4).

Chaney EM, ed. *Empowering older women: cross-cultural views.* Washington, DC, American Association of Retired Persons, 1990.

Chen BH et al. Indoor air pollution in developing countries. *World health statistics quarterly*, 1990, 43(3):127-138.

Connelly R, DeGraff DS, Levison D. *Child care policy and women's market work in urban Brazil.* Geneva, International Labour Office, 1991 (Population and Labour Policies Programme, Working Paper No. 180).

Coeytaux F, Leonard A, Royston E, eds. *Methodological issues in abortion research.* New York, The Population Council, 1989.

Darmawan J. *Rheumatic conditions in the northern part of central Java: an epidemiological survey.* West Kalimantan, Geboren te Pontianak, 1988.

de los Rios R, Gomez E. *Women in health and development: an alternative approach.* Paper prepared for the Fourth International Women's Conference, University of Rochester, New York, 10 April 1991.

Dennerstein L, Astbury J, Morse C. *Psychosocial and mental health aspects of women's health.* Geneva, World Health Organization, 1992 (unpublished document, WHO/FHE).[1]

Dixon-Mueller R, Wasserheit J. *The culture of silence. Reproductive tract infections among women in the Third World.* New York, International Women's Health Coalition, 1991.

Eaton WW et al. The incidence of specific DIS/DSM-III mental disorders: data from the NIMH epidemiological catchment area program. *Acta psychiatrica Scandinavica*, 1989, 79:163-178.

Ettling M et al. Evaluation of malaria clinics in Maesot, Thailand: use of serology to assess coverage. *Transactions of the Royal Society of Tropical Medicine and Hygiene*, 1989, 83:325-330.

Ferguson A. Women's health in a marginal area of Kenya. *Social science and medicine*, 1986, 23(1):17-29.

Gomez E. *Sex discrimination and excess female mortality among children in the Americas.* Paper prepared for the 18th NCIH International Health Conference, Arlington, VA, 23-26 June 1991.

Hertzman C. *Environment and health in Czechoslovakia.* Washington, DC, World Bank, 1990 (Internal report).

Hertzman C. *Poland: health and environment in the context of socioeconomic decline.* Washington, DC, World Bank, 1990 (Internal report).

Khan ME, Tamang AK, Patel B. Work pattern of women and its impact on health and nutrition - some observations from the urban poor. *Journal of family welfare*, 1990, 36(2):3-22.

Kickbusch I et al. *Healthy public policy: report on the Adelaide Conference.* 2nd International Conference on Health Promotion, Adelaide, 5-9 April 1988.

Koblinsky M, Gay J, Timyan J, eds. *The health of women: a global perspective.* Boulder, CO, Westview Press, forthcoming publication.

Pan American Health Organization. *Epidemiological profile of women's health in the Region of the Americas.* Washington, DC, PAHO, 1990 (unpublished document PAHO/PWD available on request from the Pan American Health Organization, 525, 23rd Street, NW, Washington, DC 20037, USA).

Royston E, Armstrong S. *Preventing maternal deaths.* Geneva, World Health Organization, 1989.

Sadik N. *Investing in women: the focus of the '90s.* New York, United Nations Population Fund (undated).

Sadik N. *The state of world population 1991.* New York, United Nations Population Fund, 1991.

De Schryver A, Meheus A. Epidemiology of sexually transmitted diseases: the global picture. *Bulletin of the World Health Organization*, 1990, 68(5):639-654.

---

[1] Unpublished WHO documents are available from the World Health Organization, 1211 Geneva 27, Switzerland. Kindly indicate document number in your request.

Selwyn BJ. The epidemiology of acute respiratory tract infection in young children: comparison of findings from several developing countries. *Reviews of infectious diseases*, 1990, 12 (supplement 8):S870-S888.

Senapati SK. *Women's work pattern and its impact on health and nutrition.* Paper prepared for the 18th NCIH International Health Conference, 23-26 June 1991, Arlington, VA.

Smith KR. *Biofuels, air pollution and health - a global review.* New York, Plenum Press, 1987,

Smyke P. *Women and health.* London, Zed Books Ltd, 1991.

Stanley K, Stjernsward J, Koraltchouk V. Women and cancer. *World health statistics quarterly*, 1987, 40(3):267-278.

Task Force for Child Survival. *Protecting the world's children: a call for action.* Proceedings of the Fourth International Child Survival Conference, 1-3 March 1990, Bangkok.

United Nations Children's Fund. *Children and women in India. A situation analysis 1990.* New Delhi, 1991.

United Nations Children's Fund. *Sex differences in child survival and development.* Amman, Jordan, United Nations Children's Fund, Regional Office for the Middle East and North Africa, 1990 (Evaluation Series No. 6).

United Nations Development Programme. *Human development report 1990.* New York, Oxford University Press, 1990.

United Nations. *The sex and age distribution of population, 1990 revision.* New York, 1990.

United Nations. *The world's women 1970-1990. Trends and statistics.* New York, 1991 (Social Statistics and Indicators, Series K, No. 8).

United Nations. *UN World Population Prospects 1990.* New York, United Nations, Department of International Economic and Social Affairs, 1991.

United Nations. *Women and nutrition.* ACC/SCN Symposium Report. Geneva, United Nations Administrative Committee on Coordination – Subcommittee on Nutrition, 1990 (Nutrition Policy Discussion Paper No. 6).

Wasserheit J. Significance and scope of reproductive tract infections among Third World women. *International journal of gynaecology and obstetrics*, 1989 suppl. (3):145-168.

World Health Organization. *Current and future dimensions of the HIV/AIDS pandemic: a capsule summary.* Geneva, 1992 (unpublished document WHO/GPA/RES/SFI/92.1).[1]

World Health Organization. *Infertility: A tabulation of available data on prevalence of primary and secondary infertility.* Geneva, 1991 (unpublished document WHO/MCH/91.9).[1]

World Health Organization. *Obstetric fistulae. A review of available information.* Geneva, 1991 (unpublished document WHO/MCH/MSM/91.5).[1]

World Health Organization. New estimates of maternal mortality. *Weekly epidemiological record*, 1991, 66(47):345-348.

World Health Organization. Prevalence of nutritional anaemia in women in the world. Geneva, 1992 (unpublished document WHO/MCH/MSM/92.2).[1]

World Health Organization. *Women and tobacco.* Geneva, 1992.

World Health Organization. *World health statistics annual 1985.* Geneva, 1986.

[1] Unpublished WHO documents are available from the World Health Organization, 1211 Geneva 27, Switzerland. Kindly indicate document number in your request.